Strength Training for Seniors

Restore Muscle With a Simple and Safe 10-Week At-Home Workout

Mark Kemp

© **Copyright 2022 - All rights reserved.**

The content contained within this book may not be reproduced, duplicated or transmitted without direct written permission from the author or the publisher.

Under no circumstances will any blame or legal responsibility be held against the publisher, or author, for any damages, reparation, or monetary loss due to the information contained within this book, either directly or indirectly.

Legal Notice:

This book is copyright protected. It is only for personal use. You cannot amend, distribute, sell, use, quote or paraphrase any part, or the content within this book, without the consent of the author or publisher.

Disclaimer Notice:

Please note the information contained within this document is for educational and entertainment purposes only. All effort has been executed to present accurate, up to date, reliable, complete information. No warranties of any kind are declared or implied. Readers acknowledge that the author is not engaged in the rendering of legal, financial, medical or professional advice. The content within this book has been derived from various sources. Please consult a licensed professional before attempting any techniques outlined in this book.

By reading this document, the reader agrees that under no circumstances is the author responsible for any losses, direct or indirect, that are incurred as a result of the use of the information contained within this document, including, but not limited to, errors, omissions, or inaccuracies.

Table of Contents

INTRODUCTION 1
   WHAT'S IN IT FOR YOU? 2
   MEET THE AUTHOR 4
   WHAT TO EXPECT 5

CHAPTER 1: IT'S TIME TO TAKE CONTROL OF YOUR LIFE 9
   WHAT'S HAPPENING TO YOUR BODY? 9
      As Your Heart Grows Older 10
      Bones, Joints, and Muscles 12
      Your Digestive System 14
      The Importance of Strengthening for Seniors 16
      Strength Training's Benefits 18

CHAPTER 2: ALL ABOUT STRENGTH TRAINING 22
   THE BASICS OF BUILDING MUSCLES, STRENGTH, ENDURANCE 22
      What is Strength Training? 23
      Specific Adaptations: SAID 24
      How Many; How Much? 25
      Positive Benefits for Seniors 28

CHAPTER 3: STRENGTH TRAINING SAFELY 34
   SAFETY IS YOUR TOP PRIORITY 34
      The Overview 35
      Important Safety Tips 37

CHAPTER 4: NUTRITIONAL STRENGTH 46
   THE PRINCIPLES OF NUTRITION 46
      Nutritional Requirements for Seniors 47
      Nutrition and Strength 48
      Nutrition Basics 49

CHAPTER 5: YOUR ANATOMY 59

WHAT YOUR MUSCLES DO AND HOW THEY WORK 59
   Muscle Anatomy 59
   Benefits of Exercises to Your Health 63
   Ergonomics: Psychological and Cognitive 65
   Your Brain and Muscle Connections 66
   Joints and Pain 68

CHAPTER 6: YOUR DIET PLAN 73

   ADD LIFE TO YOUR YEARS; ADD YEARS TO YOUR LIFE 73
   Tips for a Healthy Diet 74
   The Mediterranean Diet 78
   How To: Mediterranean Diet in Action 80
   Mediterranean Daily Menu Planning 83
   NIA Daily Menu Planning 86

CHAPTER 7: THE BASIC EXERCISES 91

   YOU CAN START AT HOME TODAY 91
   Basic Bodyweight Exercises 92

CHAPTER 8: THE DUMBBELL EXERCISES 112

   GREATER RESISTANCE FOR GREATER RESULTS 112
   Hypertrophy 112
   How Often to Lift 115
   Use It or Lose It 115
   Repetition Maximum 117
   The Dumbbell Exercises 118

CHAPTER 9: LIFTING METHODS AND TIPS 130

   MORE WAYS TO BUILD MUSCLE AND GROW STRONGER 130
   Additional Lifting Methods 130
   Method #1: Resistance Bands 131
   Method #2: Isometrics 135
   Method #3: Deadlifts 137
   Method #4: Barbells 139
   Strength Training Tips 141

CHAPTER 10: THE 10-WEEK PLAN 144

   PLANNING WILL MAKE THE DIFFERENCE FOR YOU 144
   Reps and Sets 145
   Weekly Schedules 146
   Total Body Schedule 158

CHAPTER 11: STRENGTH TRAINING FAQS	**162**
GAIN CONFIDENCE WITH KNOWLEDGE	162
CONCLUSION	**168**
THIS IS YOUR TIME: USE IT WELL	168
SUCCEED WITH PATIENCE AND CAUTION	169
SHARE THE SPIRIT	170
REFERENCES	**172**
IMAGE REFERENCES	178

Introduction

It's never too late to start. It's always too late to wait.
—Jeff Olson, visionary entrepreneur

When did you first realize that you're not as strong and physically fit as you used to be? It may have been when you were carrying a suitcase or bags of groceries, or when trying to open a jar. Maybe it was when you climbed a flight of stairs, and felt your thighs throbbing on the last few steps. You may have tried a yoga class, and couldn't keep up with the younger participants, or even the other seniors. What's going on?

Age makes no exceptions. In exchange for the years we've lived, nature exacts a price of diminishing muscle mass, reduced circulation, slower metabolism, and less energy:

- Have you reached that time in life when your physical condition has become a concern? Are you aware of the relationship between exercise and your health, but don't know what to do about it?

- Has your strength diminished, and you find it harder to lift and carry things? Are your legs no longer carrying you forward, or letting you hike or cycle effortlessly?

- Are you a man or woman over the age of 60, who is experiencing issues with your balance and mobility? Have you fallen, or are at risk of falling?

- Do you feel it's time to take charge of your life and regain the vitality and bounce that you once had, but don't know how to get started, or even what to do?

If your answer is yes, you have come to this book at the right time. It's a complete guide for all seniors who recognize that it's time to shape up, rebuild physical strength, and improve your overall health; it's a 10-week strength and fitness program that you can follow at home, or even when traveling. It will get you going and keep you going!

This is the only book you will need to regain much of that lost youth as you develop a healthier lifestyle and become stronger and in better cardiovascular condition. Through medically-approved ways to exercise and diet, you will become more fit and healthier; you will feel good, and you will look good.

What's In It For You?

What are some of the health and well-being issues that are troubling you? If you're like most seniors, these may seem familiar:

- You lack energy, and feel your strength has been slipping away as you age.

- You know you should be exercising, but don't know where to begin, or how.

- You are concerned that you may be too old for strength training, and think you might injure yourself.

- You see other people of your generation who work out, and you feel a twinge of envy, wondering why you can't be more like them.

- You are confused by the endless stream of dietary and nutritional advice coming at you on TV and online, and don't know what to trust or believe.

So how can this book turn things around for you? Here's what you will gain and why it will get you going physically, and keep you going to reach goals you had only dreamed about, and now can become real:

- **Insights.** You will understand what strength training really is, why it works, and discover all the positive things it can do for your body and your health.

- **Instructions.** You will be taught, step-by-step, how and when to perform the basic exercises that will be the most effective in strengthening and conditioning you.

- **Improvements.** The training you will receive will be a roadmap for you to follow to achieve stronger muscles, greater overall condition, and make your life better, without risking injury as you become physically fit.

- **Convenience.** Your training will focus on simple yet highly effective exercises that can be done at home, with little or minimal equipment., using your body weight for resistance. There is also training you can do with weights, if you wish and have access to dumbbells and barbells.

- **Holistic.** You will learn the importance of diet and nutrition, to increase your strength and agility, manage your weight, and protect your health and longevity. You will learn what those who live the healthiest and longest know and do.

Meet the Author

Mark Kemp is a physical therapist, nutrition expert, and the author of recently-published *Stretching for Seniors*. He is sharply focused on health in retirement, and it is this interest that fuels his enthusiasm for writing to empower seniors who want to delay, or even reverse, the aging process.

During his long professional career working with clients in all age groups, Mark has been frustrated by the fitness industry's focus on the younger generation. He believes that physical training targeted specifically at older adults can have a huge impact on their quality of life, and his goal is to help seniors to access this training independently.

Mark's credentials as an advisor on exercise for seniors are built on the substantial amount of time he spent volunteering in retirement communities, where he realized he could share his expertise and give seniors the skills they need to live more comfortably.

Recognizing how stretched staff were, he volunteered to run strength and flexibility classes for residents, and also offered nutritional advice according to individual needs.

He has continued this work throughout his career with both younger retirees and those more advanced in years, and believes it's one of the most valuable things he has to offer the world.

Mark has seen the enormous impact strength training can have in older communities and has written this book to share this information on a wider scale. He has used all the years in his experience to share this information with you in the right way

Mark lives in the UK with his wife and two dogs. He loves hiking, climbing, and cooking, and enjoys spending a Saturday outdoors before coming home to let his imagination run wild in the kitchen.

What to Expect

Strength Training for Seniors is organized into 11 chapters that will give you all you need to get into the shape and state of fitness you've been wanting, but haven't known how to begin, and do it right and do it safely:

1. Motivation: Getting started on a fitness program that will enable you to take control of your body and your life; the importance of strength training for health, well-being, and longevity.

2. Strength training: What it is, and why this is the ideal time for you to get started (or restarted) on building back your lost muscle mass and strength to gain a wide range of benefits.

3. Do no harm: Getting started with strength training with a focus on safety and prevention of injury; learning how to exercise the right way for impressive results.

4. You are what you eat: The principles and basics of nutrition, and how to eat, what to eat, and how to develop a nutrition-based lifestyle to manage your weight, your health, and to optimize the results of your strength training.

5. Your muscle anatomy: Learning the location of your major muscles and their function; how the brain-muscle interconnections are affected by exercise that releases hormones to make you feel better.

6. The diet plan. How to avoid the plethora of misguided dietary advice and adopt a nutrition-centered, medically-endorsed diet to get your weight down without obsessive calorie-counting, help build muscles and turn your eating habits into positive experiences.

7. The basic exercises. Get started immediately with these simple strengthening exercises that you can perform at home, without equipment, using your own bodyweight for resistance. You can try all 26 or focus on the ones that you want to try first, and graduate to the others when you feel ready.

8. Dumbbell exercises. Now you can move up a notch from bodyweight calisthenics to increased resistance using dumbbells. This chapter will introduce you to 15 exercises that will help you to achieve total body strengthening, and help you to understand how resistance training plus rest builds muscle mass.

9. Strength training tips. There's much more to strength and muscle building, including resistance stretching bands and isometrics—both can be done at home—plus deadlifts and barbells. There are nine essential tips to ensure best results and be injury-free.

10. 10-day plans. A good plan and checklist will get your strength training underway, with no wondering where to begin, and will keep you going for the first 10 days. You'll follow a pattern of upper body work on day 1, lower body on day 2, and rest on day 3. The plans are fully customizable to your training needs.

11. Strength training FAQs. Invariably questions will arise, no matter how comprehensive the preceding chapters have been. You may have doubts about whether strength training is something you really need, or if it's too hard, or might wonder how often you should train, and what exercises are best for you. Here's where to find the answers.

Are you ready? If you are excited about entering the first day of a new, healthier, more vibrant life, turn now to the first chapter, which will give you a motivational beginning and give you, as a senior, a better idea of why you need to embody strength training, and understand what is happening to your body.

Chapter 1:

It's Time to Take Control of Your Life

What's Happening to Your Body?

> *If not now, when? If not me, then who?*
> —Hillel the Elder, 1st Century Scholar

Welcome to the first day of the rest of your life!

This is a great beginning of the journey you are finally embarking upon because you can regain much of the strength and energy of a younger person. Let's face it, time is not a friend when it comes to our bodies, but that doesn't mean you should give up and let the universe take its toll.

In this chapter, you will gain the information and motivation you need to start strength training; to get off that couch and put the aging process into reverse gear. Let's go!

As Your Heart Grows Older

Your heart has been working hard for you all your life, bringing life-giving oxygen to every one of the trillions of cells throughout your body, nonstop, 24/7. That's quite a workout for the heart muscle, or myocardium, and inevitably, over time, those 84,000 heartbeats every day of your life really add up. No wonder things are slowing down as the years accumulate.

You probably know the basics of what your heart does, but in quick summary:

- Your heart is a **2-sided pump** that delivers oxygen in your blood to every cell in your body. As you may know, you can live for weeks without food, and days without water, but you can only live for minutes without oxygen. Your heart's essential, life-giving job is to keep the oxygen flowing throughout your body, and eliminating cellular waste.

First, how does the oxygen get into your blood? The air you inhale contains oxygen, and inside your lungs are tiny pockets—alveoli—where thin-walled capillaries absorb the oxygen atoms, allowing them to flow freely in the bloodstream, where they interact with the red blood cells.

Inside these red cells are hemoglobin proteins containing iron atoms, which bond readily with the oxygen. When the red cells reach the tissues where the oxygen is needed, the oxygen is released, and carbon dioxide ($CO2$) and other metabolic wastes are picked up by the red cells. The pressure created by your pumping heart sends the deoxygenated blood back to your heart.

The right side of your heart receives the blood on its return from the body through the veins, and pumps that blood to your lungs, where it releases the CO_2 and cellular wastes as you exhale, and receives a new supply of oxygen, as you inhale.

The oxygen-rich blood continues back to the left side of your heart, where it is received by the left atrium, then pumped through valves into the left ventricle, which gives the blood a good squeeze to send most of it—the ejection fraction—out into the aorta to begin its journey through the larger arteries and then increasingly smaller arteries and capillaries to the cells, to deliver the oxygen and complete the cycle.

So far, so good, it's an incredible process, but all those years of relentless pumping take a toll in wear-and-tear. One of the most common symptoms of aging is the stiffening of the arteries, veins, and even the small capillaries, making it harder for the blood to flow freely.

Being a muscle, your heart responds to the hard work by thickening its walls. Later, we'll get into *hypertrophy*, and how it repairs and rebuilds muscle fibers—a good thing for your skeletal muscles, but not so good for your heart, because the thickening makes it harder for the heart to pump efficiently:

- The thickened walls of the left ventricle may reduce the amount of blood it can hold and that can be delivered to the aorta.

- The valves in the heart that controls blood flow can thicken and stiffen, allowing some of the blood to flow from the ventricles backwards into the atria, causing murmurs that are common among seniors.

- The walls of the aorta and the arteries may thicken and become less flexible, which can lead to high blood pressure and increased risk of stroke.

- Over time, the reduced abilities to deliver sufficient blood and oxygen to the body can lead to heart failure, characterized by a marked reduction in energy and mobility.

Other symptoms of an aging heart include a slowing pulse rate, as the sinoatrial node, a bundle of nerves which are the heart's natural pacemaker, deteriorates, and the vagus nerve that transmits impulses from the brain to this pacemaker develops fibrous tissues and fat deposits, which can cause malfunctions include atrial fibrillation—a runaway heartbeat—and arrhythmia, which is an irregular heartbeat.

These conditions are typical, but not predestined and inevitable:

- The deterioration of a senior's heart and cardiovascular system may be slowed, suspended, and even reversed, through exercise, diet, and other lifestyle changes.

- A primary mission of this book is to help you make the changes that will not only make you stronger, but will help you to live better, and live longer.

Bones, Joints, and Muscles

Your bones, which form the skeletal structure that holds you up, will tend to shrink, become less durable, and less dense; the increased porosity known as osteoporosis. These conditions make your bones more susceptible to fractures, which becomes concerning in light of an increased susceptibility of falling as we age.

You may discover that you are no longer as tall as you used to be, as your spinal discs deteriorate and compress. You may lose even more height as your posture changes, and a condition called kyphosis causes forward bending.

Your joints are composed of bone and muscle, plus ligaments, tendons, and cushioning bursa and synovial fluids and membranes. Over time, the cushioning tissues lose their fluid, and the connective tissues lose strength, flexibility, and resilience.

Your joints also depend on cartilage, a shiny, smooth substance that coats the ends of the bones in your joints to provide lubricity needed for articulation of the joint; with time and activity, the cartilage can abrade and wear away, especially in your knees, causing pain going up and down stairs.

In addition, osteoarthritis causes calcium and other minerals to build up in your joints, limiting their range of motion, and causing stiffness and pain.

Your muscles are tissues that are constantly renewing themselves to recover from activity—the rebuilding process known as hypertrophy—but while this may balance out when you're young, it becomes more of a losing catchup game as you get older, and more muscle tissue is lost than rebuilt.

- The result: gradual loss of muscle mass, and corresponding reductions in strength, flexibility, and endurance. These, in turn, can diminish your stability, coordination, and balance, increasing the likelihood of falling, and breaking a bone!

But just as with your heart, diet, certain types of exercise, and other lifestyle changes can significantly reduce the risks of deteriorating muscles, bones, and joints. As you continue to read, you will recognize the commonality of the benefits these practices contribute to protecting and strengthening your entire body.

Your Digestive System

The stomach, the small and large intestines, the liver; these come to mind when discussing the digestive system; how your body processes and assimilates food. So let's start by thinking about the role of food in your life. We eat to stay alive, of course, but our conscious relationship with food is mostly about satisfying hunger, and the enjoyment of eating.

We're also conscious of nutrition and calories, and about protein, carbohydrates, and fats, which are the three fundamental food groups, and define everything we eat:

- **Protein** is what you may associate with building muscles and gaining strength, and that's correct, since protein is the building block of your body. From your muscles to your organs, and down to every microscopic cell, protein is what they're made of. Meat, fish, and dairy are the primary sources; plant-sourced foods are a secondary but valuable source of protein as well.

- **Carbohydrates** often get a bad rap, but they are the fuel your body runs on; the energy that keeps your heart pumping, which keeps you breathing, enables you to move, and allows the 100 billion neurons in your brain to interact and keep everything going. But carbohydrates vary in their source and quality, as you'll see later in the chapter on nutrition.

- **Fats and oils** (which are fats in liquid form) are also a source of energy, but in concentrated form, which is stored in your body for reserve, when carbohydrates are depleted. You need fats in your diet for nutritional needs, but there are good fats, like olive oil, which is primarily a heart-healthy monounsaturated fat, and bad fats, especially saturated fats which contribute to artery-clogging plaque deposits.

Now, what happens to that food you eat? You chew and swallow the food—which is mixed with saliva containing pre-digestive enzymes—travels down your esophagus to your stomach, where further enzymes and acids go to work to break down the food.

Your stomach is one place where the aging process causes trouble, as stomach acids can back up into the esophagus and cause indigestion, or, if acute, gastroesophageal reflux disease, or GERD.

Through muscular contractions, the food then passes into the small intestine where some of the food is sufficiently reduced to the molecular level, and can be absorbed into the bloodstream for eventual delivery to the cells. Food not yet sufficiently broken down to be absorbed and metabolized, continues via further contractions to the large intestine, or colon, where the trillions of beneficial bacteria in the microbiome breakdown complex carbohydrates (mostly fiber) for absorption and metabolism.

More trouble: The intestines are where constipation is caused, as the forming waste does not have adequate water or fiber to "keep things moving." Constipation is common among seniors, whose fluid intake is low or diet is unbalanced. Medications, including iron supplements and diuretics can also contribute to constipation, as can diabetes and other medical conditions.

A lack of exercise can be a contributing factor; strengthening exercises, especially those that work and condition the abdominal muscles can help improve regularity.

The Importance of Strengthening for Seniors

Whether we like it or not, as we age, we diminish a little more each year. It's part of the natural process of aging, and if left unchecked, can be inevitable: But it doesn't have to be, if you work on restoring yourself physically.

First, let's look at what's going on. You may recognize some of these consequences of the years going by.

Your metabolism slows down. This means that every process in your body, from your heartbeat and respiration, digestion and assimilation, down to the formation of proteins and production of energy in your cells; they all lose some of their vitality, and work at a slower pace.

Muscle mass and strength decrease. This is due in part to less physical activity as you get older, especially less heavy lifting and other forms of resistance exercise. It is also due to less effective repair and replacement of damaged or worn out muscle fibers, which is why seniors need more days of rest between resistance training workouts.

Body fat increases. If your daily consumption of foods remains the same over the years, but you are less active, and your metabolism has slowed, you will burn fewer calories than you ingest, and it's inevitable that the excess calories will be stored as fat. It will show up on your waistline, so keeping an eye on that by measuring the inches (or centimeters) is a good way to tell if you need to eat less, and exercise more.

Your bones: reduced density; increased porosity. Bones form the architectural structure of your body and protect what's inside; the skull protecting the brain being the most important example. Bones are made primarily of calcium, and as we age, our need for calcium increases, or, as mentioned above, your bones lose density and become more porous (less solid), and more subject to breaking. Exercise helps keep bones strong too; another advantage of building muscular strength.

Joints stiffen. We mentioned this too earlier; As you age, the bursa and other cushioning tissues in and around the joints lose their fluid, and the connective ligaments and tendons lose strength, flexibility, and resilience. The cartilage that helps lubricate joints gets worn away; runner's knee being a classic example. As a result, joints lose their range of motion, and can be painful.

Slower reflexes and reaction times. Dr. Anthony Komaroff, a professor of medicine at the Harvard Medicine School, says that "A person's reflexes and coordination become slower with age. This often leads to poor balance and slower reaction time," causing seniors to take more time to react and be more likely to stumble. This is due to "Physical changes in the nerve fibers that slow the conduction speed," according to the University of Rochester Medical Center (Reference, 2020).

Aerobic capacity decreases. Physiologists measure VO2 max, or the maximum amount of oxygen your lungs can process. This capacity is moderate to high when you're young, and especially if you are athletic and intensely active; but with the years, your lungs cannot process the intake of oxygen as efficiently, and your heart's ability to pump the oxygen-containing blood throughout your body is reduced as the heart muscle and arteries stiffen and thicken.

All of these aging phenomena are not necessarily predestined; you can take action to slow or stop the physical deterioration of your body by getting into, and staying in, good physical condition, as the following section illustrates.

Strength Training's Benefits

Preventing Injuries

As we enter "senior territory" we become increasingly susceptible to injuries. The loss of bone density—osteoporosis—can lead to bone fractures and breaks, especially if there are falls, which are common as older adults lose their sense of balance, and are less coordinated.

Osteoporosis may be treated with medication and dietary modifications, but, "There is plenty of evidence that exercise can improve bone density. Weight-bearing aerobic exercise and strength training increase density and reduce the risks of breaks" (ISSA, 2019).

Injuries among seniors go beyond bones breaking. Muscles, ligaments, and tendons can strain, pull, or tear as they lose flexibility, and ordinary lifting and carrying can do damage. And these strains and tears can happen when a fall occurs, or even when grabbing onto something to prevent a fall. But by strengthening the muscles, then the shoulders, arms, and legs can act like shock absorbers, and reduce the risk of damage being done.

Further, building strength can help reduce the likelihood of falls and stumbles, for a preemptive preventive effect.

Increasing Muscle Mass

If things feel heavier to lift these days, from a large carton of milk to a suitcase, it isn't your imagination:

- According to ISSA (2019), "By the age of 70, the average adult has lost 25 percent of muscle mass. And this is due mostly to disuse and inactivity."

It happens slowly, but gradually the size and strength of the muscles diminish. But this loss of muscle mass can be reversed: The repair and rebuilding process (hypertrophy) may be slower with age, but it remains capable of responding to the customary damage to muscle tissues caused by hard exercise, and can overbuild as it repairs, and increase muscle mass, and strength.

So when a senior begins strength training, like weightlifting, or bodyweight resistance training, this can reverse the loss and increase muscle size and tonality (firmness) and power. This positive effect depends on the regularity of exercise, graduated increments of resistance over time, and adequate rest between resistance workouts—a two or three day rest and recovery time is advised for seniors.

Improving Functional Movement

With age, our bodies stiffen and grow less flexible, as ligaments and tendons harden and reduce the range of motion of our joints. It becomes apparent as we walk and our steps are shorter, our knees ache, and our ankles don't flex. Reaching, especially over our heads, is restrained by tight shoulder joints and sore muscles. Add in the reduced muscle size and strength, and it's apparent that we aren't who we once were.

But here too, the right exercises can turn things around, increasing our flexibility, extending the range of motion of our joints, and putting more spring back into our steps. Increasing muscular strength through training is foundational for improving our functional movement. Mature adults can regain lost mobility, walk faster and farther, and even reduce the need for canes, crutches, and other assistive devices including walkers and rollators, by regularly performing strength training.

Building strength and increasing flexibility can also help with other functional movements, from rolling over in bed to getting up from a chair, or safely and more easily getting in and out of the bathtub. Our lives can become easier, and we can regain access to more of the activities we once enjoyed.

Restructuring Body Composition

Seniors tend to gain more fat at the same time they are losing muscle mass. This happens especially among women, and occurs even without weight gain, although a majority of seniors are overweight or obese. Despite what you may have heard, the muscles do not "turn to fat," but there is a reduction of muscle tissues coincidental with increasing fat cell deposits.

The downside of this restructuring goes beyond looking and feeling "soft," as the increased presence of fat increases the risk of chronic illnesses, ranging from type 2 diabetes to heart disease, and even some types of cancer.

But there's an upside: The restructuring of your body can be slowed appreciably. The right kinds of exercise can help to maintain a healthy body composition with a more moderate level of body fat, and a weight in the normal range. Strength training can be of measurable benefit in getting your body back into shape.

Benefitting Mood and Sociability

Seniors can become increasingly isolated as they become less energetic, less mobile, and more focused inward on their health, physical condition, and prospects for the future. Some may be retired, and are lacking the challenges and stimulation of work, and also are missing out on the social interaction with fellow workers, as well as with those in their community. These conditions can lead to feelings of loneliness and depression.

Strength training can change this scenario dramatically, by restoring energy, movement and mobility, and rebuilding self-confidence. When you feel stronger and in good condition, your mood improves, and you can return to being outward and interactive. You will stop worrying about yourself, and feel healthy and fit. A discouraged, negative attitude can be replaced with positivism.

A deeper dive. You've just gained an overview of what strength training can do for you, but you don't have the whole picture yet; there's much more to come. In the next chapter, we are going to dive deeper into everything there is to know about strength training and why you should incorporate it into your lifestyle.

Chapter 2:

All About Strength Training

The Basics of Building Muscles, Strength, Endurance

This chapter will give you deeper insight into what strength training really is, and how beneficial it can be for your body. It's time to let go of misunderstandings and get the facts about what strength training can do to slow, even turn back, the aging process.

Maybe you've given strength training a try at some point, and didn't see much benefit, or you felt you've left push ups and crunches in the past; that weightlifting and calisthenics are for young people. Don't be hesitant about strength training, or feel that it's intimidating, and is for others.

Yes, bodybuilders can do it, younger people can do it, but older people can do it too, and can achieve real anti-aging benefits. The beautiful thing about strength training is how it can be tailored to your body; as a type of training that is versatile, and can be adapted to your specific needs, and allow you to work safely within any limitations you may have.

As we'll explain, as a senior you will not be "bulking up" like a bodybuilder, but you can regain some of the muscle mass you've lost, so you can firm up what's become saggy, and get some good cardiovascular conditioning, as well.

What is Strength Training?

Strength training is often called resistance training, because it is a "Specialized method of conditioning that involves the progressive use of assorted resistive loads and a variety of training modalities intended to promote health, fitness, and sport specific performance," as defined in *Precision Nutrition* (Andrews, 2022).

It's called resistance training because it requires your muscles to overcome varying degrees of, well, resistance. There are different forms or methods of creating resistance, with the most common being:

- **Weights**—either free weights, like dumbbells, barbells, and kettle weights, or weight machines that you'll find at most gyms, and which use pulleys and mechanics that you pull or push to lift weights in controlled movements.

- **Bodyweight calisthenics**—using only your own weight to provide resistance, and requiring little or no equipment; push ups, pull ups, planks, leg raises, crunches, dips, and squats are among the most familiar, but there are many more.

- **Resistance bands**—these are flat rubber bands or tubes that are stretched to achieve resistance. They come in different colors based on the resistance level, and can be used at home (or anywhere) to replicate free weights, or to intensify calisthenics.

The fundamental principle of strength training is to exert or strain muscle tissue repetitively to cause a deterioration in the muscle tissues and fibers, which is subsequently repaired by the addition of new protein molecules.

The amount of protein replacement is proportional to the exertion, and if the damage is sufficient, the repair slightly overbuilds the muscle tissue, increasing muscle mass. This process is called **hypertrophy**, and over time, makes your muscles bigger and firmer.

Does this mean strength training will bulk you up like a bodybuilder? No, not unless you work out with the commitment and intensity of increasingly (very) heavy weights that a serious weightlifter has to heave. You will not turn into Arnold Schwarzenegger!

And even then, there's another limiting factor: age. As a senior, you no longer have the hormonal levels of youth, especially testosterone, which, by the way, women have as well as men, although at lower levels. Talk with your doctor before taking any hormonal supplements, and steer clear of anabolic steroids.

But don't let this discourage you! To the contrary, seniors can definitely experience the positive benefits of resistance training, as you'll see later in this chapter.

Specific Adaptations: SAID

Physiologists use the acronym SAID, which stands for "specific adaptations to imposed demands," which means that your body will tend to adapt in direct relationship to the types and intensities of demands that you impose upon them. Specifically:

- When you perform particular movements, with time and practice you will improve how you do those movements.

- When you perform a partial range of motion, you will gain strength only in that range of motion; doing a full range of motion will enable you to get stronger throughout the full range.

- When you perform resistance exercises using light weights and many repetitions in long-duration sets, you will build endurance.

- When you perform resistance exercises using medium-to-heavy weights and fewer repetitions in medium-duration sets, you will build muscle mass.

- You will also build muscle mass using even heavier weights and even fewer repetitions in shorter sets, assuming there's sufficient exercise volume to the workout.

Let's go deeper into repetitions, sets, and rest, which are the three parts of the resistance training and strength-building cycle.

How Many; How Much?

Repetitions, or reps, are the number of times you lift and lower the weight or resistance, or push up and down, or pull back and forth. When you hold dumbbells or a barbell while you are standing or sitting on a bench, and you curl (lift) the weight to your shoulders, and then lower it to the starting position; that is one rep. The same goes for the down-and-up of one push up, or the up and down of one pullup.

Sets are the group of repetitions performed during one sequence, or round. If you curl the barbell 10 times sequentially, without stopping, that is one set of 10 reps. You will normally then rest briefly (about 60 seconds for lighter weights; up to 3 minutes if you lift heavy weights, for example), or perform a different exercise for another body part, like squats or toe lifts for the legs. You would then repeat the 10 curl reps, for a second set, rest, and then do one more set of 10 reps.

Rest between sets is not a luxury; it's a necessity. Within the muscles, tiny energy factories, the mitochondria, need to recharge. It's a fascinating chemical process involving a molecule called adenosine-triphosphate (ATP), breaking and reconnecting its high energy hydrogen bonds. In just a minute, your muscles are recharged at least partially, enabling you to perform the next set.

The questions you may ask include "How many reps; how much weight or resistance?" The answers are variable, and depend on you, your physical abilities, and your ambitions; what those weights and reps should be depends on you. As noted above, if your goal is more endurance-focused, you'll want to lift a lighter weight for more reps; for muscle mass, and getting bigger muscles, then use a heavier weight for fewer reps.

Here's a simple guideline you can follow:

- You will be able to determine sufficient volume of repetitions in a set, whether using light, medium, or heavy weights by reaching enough reps that the last one or two are difficult, and it would be very hard to do more.

- For example, you might lift a 10 lb weight for 20 reps, or a 20 lb weight for 10 reps. In the first case, around rep 17 or 18 it could start to be hard to do many more.

With that 20 lb weight, your muscles would be letting you know it's tough by rep 8 or 9.

It is important to keep good posture and form, especially during the last reps in a set, when it gets tough, and you may be tempted to slouch, or fail to do the full range of motion.

How about the number of sets? Here too there are many options, but for simplicity, especially when starting your strength training, three sets is the standard, whether you're doing many or few reps per set. A rest between sets one and two, and between two and three is common practice; from 60 seconds to three minutes, depending on the heaviness of what you're using for resistance.

Can you do more than three sets? Yes, of course, that's up to you. Some who perform resistance training prefer up to 10 sets; albeit with each set not being to exhaustion. It may be best to keep it to three sets, and make each one count!

Progression can be achieved as your conditioning increases by increasing the weight or resistance, or by increasing the reps, or a bit of both. Using bicep curls with dumbbells as our example, you might begin lifting 10 lbs (each arm) for 12 reps per set, and later, when it feels comfortable in a week or two, increase the weight to 12.5 or even 15 lbs. Or, keep the weight at 10 lbs and increase the reps from 12 to 18 lbs. Or, toss a fourth set into the mix.

Feel free to experiment with weights and reps, to find the combination that works for you; it's your body, and only you can tell what feels best, and works best.

But don't try to increase your workout intensity by shortening the rest period between sets; this is a "sacred time" that your muscles need to metabolically recharge the energy stores in your mitochondria. Rest between sets for at least 60 seconds with lighter weights in an endurance workout, and up to three minutes with heavier weights for building muscle mass.

Positive Benefits for Seniors

Americans, especially city-dwellers, tend to be sedentary, and in poor shape physically. Unsurprisingly, their inactive lifestyle, and along with bad dietary habits, leads to increases in body weight.

The basic determinant of weight status is the body mass index, or BMI. It's a simple correlation of height and weight. Normal weight is in the BMI range of 18.5 to 24.9; overweight is between 25.0 and 29.9; and a BMI of 30.0 or higher is designated as obese. These readings don't take into account different physiologies, like the weight of muscle vs. fat, but are a useful guideline. You can learn your BMI by looking online for any of the free instant calculators.

Physiologist and author Dr. Wayne Westcott specializes in exercise for seniors, and notes that up to "80 percent of men and women in their 50s and older have too little muscle and too much fat, leading to obesity, osteoporosis, and diabetes." He further cites increases in "High blood pressure, high blood cholesterol, heart disease, stroke, arthritis, low back pain, and numerous types of cancer" (Human Kinetics, 2022).

Fortunately, seniors can still experience the positive benefits of resistance training: More muscle mass, greater strength and flexibility, and stronger bones. There are cardiovascular benefits too, since a good resistance workout will get you heart pumping and your blood flowing. The number of strength training benefits for you as a senior include these:

- **Cardiovascular health.** While your muscles are firming and rebuilding mass, the effort is engaging the cardiovascular and respiratory systems by creating intensified demand for oxygen-rich blood delivery. This strengthens the heart muscle and widens arteries to decrease high blood pressure, and improve aerobic capacity.

  The risks of high blood pressure, or hypertension, are appreciable, affecting about one-third of American adults. Dr. Westcott is encouraged by a number of studies that have shown "Significant reductions in resting blood pressure readings after two more months of standard or circuit-style strength training."

- **Cardio recovery.** For seniors who have already experienced cardiovascular health issues, resistance exercise has proven effective in helping them to achieve and maintain a lower, more normal body weight, along with building muscle mass and increasing strength. By improving physical performance, resistance training helps speed recovery from the heart or circulatory event, and restore independence.

- **Blood lipids.** Another key component of preventing or managing heart disease is controlling blood lipids. "Almost half of American adults have undesirable blood lipid levels, increasing their risk for heart disease," says Dr. Wescott. But consistent strength training over time can lead to "Favorable increases of 8 to 21 percent in HDL ('good') cholesterol," as well as a desirable reduction of 13 to 23 percent in LDL ('bad') cholesterol, and beneficial 11 to 18 percent reductions in triglycerides.

- **More activity.** Building muscular strength improves your ability to engage in daily activities, in addition to enhancing your strength and endurance, and your speed and agility. Resistance training can elevate your physical performance, speed up your recovery times, and make you more confident and productive.

  Your improved balance from strengthening will further enhance your agility and reduce the risk of experiencing falls, and the injuries they can cause.

- **Metabolic improvement.** Strengthening improves your metabolic rate, which takes place at the cellular level. This can help protect you from many chronic diseases and conditions, including type 2 diabetes, obesity, and, as noted above, cardiovascular disease.

  Studies report that glucose tolerance is improved and insulin sensitivity is better controlled after a few weeks of resistance training. This means that your body will be less reactive to the foods you eat, and while good dietary practices are strongly recommended, you will have greater latitude in your food choices.

  Resistance training has a positive impact on your metabolic rate by increasing your use of energy during both the resistance training session and the recovery and rebuilding of your muscles, which extend up to three days following every hard workout.

- **Fat reduction.** You understand the dangers of being overweight or obese, which can threaten your health: As we've already noted, excess body fat can lead to a number of diseases; type 2 diabetes and heart disease being the most prominent. That extra fat can also slow you down, by reducing your physical abilities, and limiting your energy.

Dr. Westcott reports that research conducted during resistance training programs noted an average gain of "Three to four pounds of muscle after just three to four months of strength training." Weight management is helped by caloric expenditure during resistance exercise; any additional weight gain from building muscle mass is more than offset by fat reduction.

- **Denser bones.** As reported in York Fitness (2022), if a person is sedentary, they can "Lose up to 4 percent bone density and 5 percent muscle mass per year after age 30." Strengthening your muscles and connective tissues increases bone density, making your bones less susceptible to breakage, and lowering the risks of injuries; as you've read, the bones of seniors can become fragile with osteoporosis.

Dr. Westcott reports that "Substantial increases in bone mineral density have been seen after several months of regular resistance exercise," adding that consistent strength training may actually be the "Most productive means for developing a strong and injury-resistant musculoskeletal system."

- **Improved coordination.** In addition to building and strengthening muscle tissue, resistance training can improve your "Intermuscular and intramuscular coordination—in other words, the ability to coordinate your moving parts" (Andrews, 2022). It also increases the strength of tendons, ligaments, and other connective tissues that join muscles to bones and joints.

Your progress can be measured by your "Improving rate of force production—how quickly you can generate force to move against the resistance."

- **Improving memory.** Studies are finding links between cognitive health and physical exercise, including resistance workouts that are performed over an extended period. Daily exercise is reversing some symptoms of memory loss among Alzheimer's patients, providing encouraging early evidence that a progressive, ongoing strength training program may be able to prevent or reduce long term memory impairment among seniors.

- **Mental health.** Finally, there are other psychological benefits of increasing strength and endurance, like enhanced self-esteem, confidence, and sense of well-being. Additionally, a good resistance workout releases the beta endorphin hormones that cause a feeling of elation, known among athletes as the "runner's high." This sense of calm and creativity can last for hours after each workout.

Strength training has been shown to reduce depression, improve physical self-concept, and help seniors to snap out of fatigue and become revitalized. The workouts have raised their sense of tranquility, lowered stress, anxiety, and tension, and encouraged positive social engagement, and elevated their overall mood.

As reported in York Fitness (2022), a study of seniors who were over age 60 and suffering from depression concluded that "Most participants assigned to a higher-intensity resistance program saw up to a 50 percent improvement in their mood and other initially reported symptoms."

Strength training workouts have been proven to be valuable to health and well-being; as you have seen, strength training has quite a few incredible benefits that can help you on many levels, from building muscle mass and lowering body fat to improving memory and mood.

Adding to these benefits are even more positives, like being able to perform resistance exercises where and when you want, especially in the convenience of your home. There's no need to invest in expensive equipment, since bodyweight calisthenics require no equipment, except an optional, inexpensive portable pull up bar. Stretch bands are also a very low cost option, and can be carried easily to use at work or when traveling.

Dumbbells, barbells, and kettle weights are a bit higher in cost, but a small set will not set you back too much, if weightlifting is your preference. And if you have access to a gym or fitness center, all the equipment you might need is there for you.

Strength training also deserves credit for providing you with a drug-free option to resolve physical and mental problems. All of the above benefits illustrate the effectiveness of building strength and endurance as ways to ease pain in your muscles and joints, and to elevate your state of mind and self-esteem. But be sure to check with your doctor regarding prescribed medications, and do not go off your meds without checking.

Coming up. In the next chapter, you will get further into the details and principles of strength training, with an emphasis on safety and avoiding injuries.

Chapter 3:

Strength Training Safely

Safety is Your Top Priority

Primum non nocere: First, do no harm.

—Hippocratic Oath

Counseling those who are new to resistance training to be careful to avoid injury is a necessity for those at any age, but is of extra importance to seniors, whose vulnerability to tears, strains, pulls, and breaks increases with age. Seniors can achieve great progress with progressive strength training, but caution and responsible practices are essential.

So as you prepare to enter the realm of resistance workouts, safety should be your top priority, and should not be overshadowed by your enthusiasm and ambition to gain strength, muscle mass, and endurance, while burning off fat.

The objective of this chapter is to help you understand how to exercise in a way that will enable you to build muscles and strengthen connective tissues without causing injuries. Take time to give these cautions your fullest attention, and you can look forward to years of steady growth and progress, without getting sidelined.

The Overview

As we get into safety and injury prevention, here's a reminder of what strength training is: It's a form of conditioning that requires your muscles to be exerted against varying degrees of resistance. That resistance is generally provided by weightlifting, bodyweight calisthenics, and more recently, rubber stretch bands and tubes.

Australia's *Better Health* (2022) sums it up as "Resistance training (also called strength training or weight training) is the use of resistance to muscular contraction to build the strength, anaerobic endurance and size of skeletal muscles." Progress depends on staying with the training over time: "Regular, repeated and consistent resistance training results in stronger muscles."

Benefits. Highlighting the benefits of strength training from the previous chapter, we're reminded they are numerous, and in addition to building muscle mass and strength, include improved cardiovascular conditioning, lower blood pressure, reduction of LDL cholesterol and triglycerides, and recovery from heart issues.

Other benefits are an improved metabolic rate; energy to be more active and engaged; reduction of fat and increased bone density; better coordination and balance; improved memory; and a better mental state and mood

Risks. But let's look before we leap, and briefly recall why a senior's body "ain't what it used to be." Joints become stiffer and may become painful as muscles, connective ligaments and tendons tighten and lose flexibility, resulting in reduced range of motion. Joints can also be constrained—and pained—by osteoarthritis.

Bones become more porous and susceptible to breakage, which can happen if weights that are lifted are too heavy, or if there are falls, due to balance issues brought on by age.

- Lesson: Do not try to keep up with others, who may be able to lift more than you can because they're younger or simply have been working out longer, and are conditioned. Stay attentive to your form and posture to counter balance issues.

- Lesson: Take it easy as your body slowly acclimates to strength training workouts; it's one thing to do sufficient reps with a weight you can handle, but it's another to overextend and lift a weight that's too much for you, and end up pulling or tearing a muscle or tendon.

The heart keeps pumping throughout our lives, but it too can stiffen, as can the arteries, veins, and capillaries, making it harder for the heart to pump efficiently, and deliver oxygen to the muscles and renew their energy.

- Lesson: Warm up before heavy lifting instead of jumping right in with a heavier weight than you can easily handle. Give your cardiovascular system time to loosen up and become more flexible and oxygenate your muscle tissues, enabling you to keep up with the workload.

Age also slows the rebuilding process—hypertrophy—that takes place after the muscles have been exerted in a hard workout, and new protein overbuilds and strengthens the damaged muscle fibers. This process takes longer the older we are.

- Lesson: Rest between resistance training workouts, so your muscles can recover. Allow at least one full day of rest; preferably two days, before exerting the same muscles. You can do resistance workouts every day, but only if you alternate muscle groups.

Rest between workouts is separate from the minute or so of rest that you need between sets; that rest is for the mitochondrial energy recharge in the muscle cells.

Important Safety Tips

Resistance training can be tremendously beneficial to seniors, but only if its risks and potential dangers are managed—which they can be, by following the proper techniques and practices. That's why it's important for you to become familiar with these safety tips; please take these cautions seriously

First, See Your Doctor

If you are to '*do no harm*' to yourself, get checked out medically. See a doctor who can conduct a pre-exercise screening to assess your current state of fitness, and especially to identify any medical conditions you may have that could risk an injury or medical event during a strength training workout.

- Avoidance of cardiovascular damage is of highest priority, and if you have previously experienced symptoms of heart disease, it would be best to be seen by your cardiologist. This is not to imply that you should not be working out; to the contrary, your heart will benefit from conditioning. But there may be some exercises that your doctor will prefer for you to practice, and some that may be advised to avoid, or practice with restraint.

- Other medical conditions that may require a medical heads up include osteoporosis, since bone damage can be a risk, especially if lifting heavy weights is involved, and also any tendencies you may have to pull or tear muscles or connective tissues. Conditions like bursitis, which is loss of cushioning fluid in the joints, may call for moderation of certain movements.

Learn the Correct Techniques

It's essential to know how to do it right! Most injuries are caused by improper lifting, bad posture, imbalance, and general carelessness. Later in this book you will learn how to perform the strengthening exercises; benefit from these instructions and reduce the risks of hurting yourself.

- The other benefit of good techniques is the results you will achieve, since your muscles will be most responsive to the optimal weights, reps, and sets, performed with the correct movements and ideal posture. In contrast, racing through the workouts carelessly, and doing the movements sloppily, will not produce good results, as well as increasing the risks of injury.

- If you have any doubts about your strengthening program, don't hesitate to seek **professional guidance**. There are many trainers who are qualified in weight training, and can select the right exercises for you, help to choose the weight levels, reps, and sets, and even keep a record of your progress. But be sure to work with a trainer who has experience working specifically with seniors. You can also find many good instructive videos online.

Proceed Slowly and Controlled

Take it easy. There's no hurry or rush when performing resistance exercises. And don't toss the weights around; keep them under control, following a precise movement path. As *Better Health* advises, "Don't throw them up and down or use momentum to 'swing' the weights through their range of motion."

- One reason is to reduce the risks of hurting yourself by lifting, pulling, or stretching too fast, which can cause damage before you realize anything's wrong. Going through the motion at a slower, more deliberate pace, and in prescribed movements, allows you to feel what's happening, and if there is a potential strain or pull likely to happen, you can react and stop before damage is done.

- Another reason to slow it down is to optimize the effects of the exercise. By bringing that weight up slowly, and by more slowly lowering that pushup, you will contract the muscles more productively. Yes, it's harder to lift or lower slowly, but that's the point, isn't it? Your muscles will respond more fully when the resistance movements are slow and deliberate, than when rushed.

- Yet another rationale for slower movement is the mental benefit of being in the moment by being fully conscious of the exercise movement, and how it feels. This focuses your concentration in a brief meditative effect, helping to lower stress and anxiety. At the end of a slow, thoughtful workout, the result will be a state of self-assurance and positivity, further augmented by the release of beta endorphin hormones.

Use Quality Equipment

If you choose to acquire weights and other resistance equipment to use at home, be selective and go for better quality, because cheap equipment can break, malfunction, and potentially cause physical damage.

- If you use the equipment in a gym or fitness center, make sure there are no damaged or broken cables, and all is in working order. If you only are using dumbbells or barbells, be sure the weights are secured, and nothing heavy can fall off while you're hoisting the object, especially when lifting over your head.

- Bodyweight calisthenics are essentially equipment free, but you need to be careful when involving furniture—like when doing triceps dips with a chair, or when steadying yourself for balance—so that you are safely supported. You may want to use a portable pullup bar, which is placed in a doorway; these devices require no installation, but can be used safely and effectively, as long as correctly positioned.

Breathe Effectively

Breathing may not be top of mind when you're performing strength training exercises, but it's important for safety as well as for optimal performance. Always exhale during the hard part of the movement; when the weight or resistance is being lifted or pushed, and inhale as you lower or release the weight. "Never hold your breath while straining," advises *Harvard Health* (2018):

- Holding your breath while lifting a heavy weight is known as the "Valsalva maneuver; it can temporarily raise your blood pressure considerably and can be risky for people with cardiovascular disease."

- Deeper, thoughtful breathing is as fundamental to strength training as to yoga and meditation because it helps you to focus your attention on the pace of the movement, while helping to deliver more oxygen to your muscles for added energy. Just as noted above, to proceed slowly with the movement, managed breathing will calm as well as energize you.

Good Posture

Form is a component of strength training, and as with proceeding slowly and performing movements the right way, good posture can help prevent the injuries that bad posture may cause, and will ensure the fullest benefit from the exercise.

- When reading the instructions for the strengthening exercises, be attentive to how you should position your body and place the weight before starting the movement, whether standing, sitting, or lying on a bench or the floor.

- Control your posture during the movement too, to prevent placing extra pressure on your spine; both the upper and lower back are susceptible to strains, especially when your back needs to be upright, not bent.

- **Bend joints.** Another form-related issue: *Harvard Health* recommends "Don't lock your joints; always leave a slight bend in your knees and elbows when straightening out your legs and arms."

When Sick or Injured

There are times when you need to take it easy: when you are sick; when you are injured; and when you are simply exhausted (for any number of reasons, including a bad night's sleep, or following a difficult travel experience). Protecting your health is of paramount importance, and you do not want to overextend yourself.

- Be especially careful not to aggravate an injury by putting the muscles or joint under physical strain, since that can turn a minor problem into a major, potentially debilitating injury. Your body won't mind if you miss a few workouts; in fact, extra rest means longer recovery time, allowing the muscles to repair and rebuild.

- You can continue strength training while injured if you can avoid engaging the injured area, muscles, or joints. For example, a strain in your shoulder and upper arm will preclude working the upper body, but you can perform exercises for the core, glutes, and legs if the arms and shoulders are not involved.

The Power of Rest

We've talked about the essential role of rest between workouts, but it's worth revisiting to emphasize the importance of rest, and why it's key to building strength, muscle mass, and endurance. You need to appreciate that these results are due to a process of destruction and rebuilding of muscle tissue: hypertrophy.

- The exertion that your muscles go through during a good resistance workout causes some damage to the cells; they're working overtime to provide the energy your muscles need to contract and lift heavy objects. Rest is required to allow them to rebuild.

- As *Healthline* (2019) sums it up, "To build muscle through weight lifting, you need to have both mechanical damage and metabolic fatigue." This generally causes structural damage and mechanical damage to muscle proteins that "Stimulates a repair response in the body. The damaged fibers in muscle proteins result in an increase in muscle size."

- Hypertrophy sends new protein molecules to repair, and slightly overbuilds the damaged muscle cells. But only if *sufficient rest* is accorded to those muscles.

- **How much rest?** At least one day of rest between hard workouts, and ideally two days, or even three for seniors, whose recovery times are longer. So for full body workouts, plan on strength training two or three days a week, at most, to ensure adequate rest.

- But you can do your resistance workout more often—even daily—if you alternate body regions and muscle groups, e.g., chest, arms, and shoulders on day one; core on day two; and legs on day three, then optionally rest for a day, and then repeat the cycle.

Warm Up and Cool Down

First, warm up. This goes for all types of vigorous exercise, but especially for strength training. Before starting the heavy lifting, pulling, and pushing, your muscles, connective tendons, and ligaments are not yet flexible, nor are they rich with oxygen. In this state, they are more susceptible to strains or other problems. Further, the muscles are at their low point of strength, so jumping right into the workout will make the movements more difficult; the weights will feel heavier, and you'll have to work harder.

- But be careful not to try to warm up by performing intensive stretching, since cold muscles and connective tissues don't appreciate that either, and there are risks of injury.

- An ideal, safe warmup is to do a cardio (aerobic) workout first, since it will get your blood and oxygen flowing to all parts of your body, and get your heart and breathing rates elevated. Depending on your preferences, this can be a brisk 10 minute walk, followed by some *light* stretching, or your full 30 minute or longer cardio workout for the day. You can also warm up by lifting lighter than your usual weights.

- **Cooling down** after strength training is when it's time to do the stretching, since everything is well warmed up and flexible, and receptive to being stretched for even greater flexibility. Be sure to stretch the muscle groups you've just exercised. A round of yoga stretches can provide a good range of movements.

Manage Expectations

It's okay to look forward to building muscles and getting stronger, but be realistic. Don't expect to feel and see significant improvements within days; this is more of a marathon, so to speak, than a sprint. You may make progress after each workout, but it's imperceptible on a day-to-day basis, so don't be impatient and end up overexerting yourself. Give it time, and your efforts will pay off.

- A more immediate effect you can expect is the temporary increase in muscle size and tone that you may experience for a brief period after a hard resistance training workout. This is caused by an accumulation of blood in the muscle tissues that brought the needed oxygen and nutrients. Your muscles will feel tight and firm until the excess blood subsides after an hour or two.

Obey Your Body

Our final tip is for you to listen to your body; do not ignore its signals that something may be wrong, and you need to ease up, or stop the exercise immediately. Be especially alert to pain, which can be a warning that a muscle or connective tissue is starting to strain or tear.

- It's not a concern if you feel fatigue or near-exhaustion, especially during the last few reps of a set, but a sharp pain is definitely a concern you need to respond to. You can reduce the weight or level of resistance and try again, but if the pain persists, call it quits for the day for that muscle group. If the pain persists for more than a few days, you may need to get it checked out medically.

Next: nutrition. The quality of your diet can directly influence the effects of your strength training as well as your overall health, and even your longevity. Diet and nutrition are what we'll cover next, to give you a clear path to self-optimization.

Chapter 4:

Nutritional Strength

The Principles of Nutrition

Strength training does not exist in a vacuum, independent of other factors; its partner in building muscles and making you stronger is nutrition. The expression, "You are what you eat," is fundamentally correct because what we ingest becomes the building blocks of cellular growth and our sources of energy; understanding nutrition is an essential part of your learning process, and should become integrated into your lifestyle as you train.

Going further, good nutrition is critically important to your health, and affects not only how well you live, but also how long you live. It's surprising how few people take nutrition seriously, or take the trouble to understand it. This chapter, and the following, will arm you with the knowledge you need to optimize your physical potential.

Good nutrition involves eating foods that provide a complete and balanced source of the essential food groups—complex carbohydrates, proteins, and healthy fats/oils—along with the vitamins, minerals, and other nutrients that help your body to effectively digest and metabolize the foods you eat.

As defined by the National Institute of Health in *Medline Plus* (2022), "Nutrients are substances in foods that our bodies need so they can function and grow."

Nutritional Requirements for Seniors

Good nutrition is important for everyone at any age, for health and vitality, and to manage weight, but it becomes particularly important as we age, because our needs change. For example, a senior's metabolic rate may change, and fewer calories are needed to maintain a normal weight, yet there is a need for certain nutrients that should not be reduced.

Some seniors may need more protein in their diet, especially if they are trying to build muscle mass. But there are nutritional requirements for seniors, apart from exercise related needs. There are certain lifestyle and situational changes that can occur as we age, and which may make it difficult for seniors to eat nutritionally. These include:

- Isolation, which can happen when an older person is living alone, or becomes less mobile and unable to shop for foods, and to prepare and cook for themselves. This can also be the result of health issues, and can result in a dependency on prepared meals that may be low in nutrients, and high in undesirable saturated fats, sodium and sugar.

- Medicines may change the taste of food, cause dry mouth, or diminish appetite, causing insufficient consumption of nutritious foods. Other side effects from drugs and medications may be fatigue, disorientation, imbalance, and nausea.

- Reduced or lower income, which may happen in retirement, and possibly lead to a reduced budget for food. A person who has preferred more natural foods may have to give those up, and may have to select more mass produced, processed foods.

- Aging can reduce a person's senses of taste and smell, thus lowering their appetite. There can also be difficulty chewing and swallowing, and frequent indigestion, or acid reflux.

Nutrition and Strength

Good nutrition is needed for good health, as you know, but it has particular importance when you are participating in resistance training to build muscle mass and increase strength and endurance.

Weightlifting, bodyweight calisthenics, and using stretch bands for resistance take a toll on our bodies, causing damage to tissues, as well as expending large amounts of energy. Nutrition is what will help to rebuild damaged muscle tissues, by supplying sufficient protein; nutrition will also be pivotal in restoring the depleted energy stored in cells by supplying carbohydrates for more immediate use, and storing fats, to keep energy in reserve.

But as you will see, the sources of proteins, carbohydrates, and fats vary widely in their quality and even safety relative to our health:

- Nutritious protein is obtained from lean meat, fish, low-fat dairy, and eggs, as well as partially from whole grains, seeds, and nuts. The animal sources of protein need to be low in saturated fats, and most plant-based protein is incomplete, meaning they need to be combined, like rice and beans, or served with animal protein.

- Healthy carbohydrates are complex, meaning they retain their nutrients like vitamins, minerals, and fiber; they are slower to digest and metabolize than refined cereals and sugars, so do not cause a spike in blood sugar and a strong insulin response. Complex, nutritional carbs are found in vegetables, fruits, whole grains, beans, nuts, and seeds.

- Fats are needed for nutrients as well as a source of reserved energy. One issue with fats and oils (liquid fats) is their high calorie concentration (more than double, per gram, than protein and carbs).

Many fats are high in saturates, which are conducive to heart disease; the medically-endorsed sources are extra virgin olive oil and avocados, which are high in heart-healthy monounsaturates. The fats in cold water fish are also highly beneficial, being low in saturates, and high in omega-3 fatty acids, which have antioxidant properties.

Nutrition Basics

The Canadian government's *Food Guide* (2022) sums up the unique nutritional needs of seniors:

- "Healthy eating is a key part of aging well. It is a way for you to stay healthy and strong, which is important to maintain your independence and quality of life."

Healthy eating is necessary to help protect and promote your health and well-being by providing the essential nutrients and energy your body needs to keep you going. Good nutrition can help lower the risk of chronic diseases, including heart disease, and type 2 diabetes.

You can also prevent bone loss caused by osteoporosis (bone porosity and weakness, which we've covered earlier) to reduce your risk of breaking bones due to falling.

Managing Your Weight

Maintaining a normal weight is at the top of most priorities for health at any age, but especially for seniors. As we age, our metabolic rate slows, so we burn fewer calories during the day than we used to, and the leftover calories are stored as fat. We also tend to be less active and more sedentary; we don't walk as often or as far as we used to, and sit for longer stretches. When this coincides with continuation of our usual eating behavior, gradual weight gain is inevitable; here's why:

- The concept of "calories in; calories out" means there is no way around the simple principle that extra calories must be accounted for, generally as fat. If you want to lose weight, you need to eat less, and exercise more. This does not mean having to starve yourself, or deprive yourself of what you enjoy; nor does it require exhaustive daily workouts

- Moderation is key, and you will discover that you can adjust your eating behavior and adopt a totally enjoyable dietary plan, and increase your physical activity gradually.

- How do you determine if your weight is normal? Refer back to Chapter 1's explanation of the BMI; the body mass index, which is based on your height and weight. Normal weight is in the BMI range of 18.5 to 24.9; over that is overweight, or obese, and putting you at risk for type 2 diabetes and heart disease.

Shopping and Cooking

Some senior adults may live within a large, multigenerational family environment, and don't have to be concerned about planning and preparing meals. But for seniors who live alone, or with just one other, grocery shopping and cooking can be challenging.

If this sounds like your own situation, take a little time to plan. Decide what you like, and consider modifications to introduce healthier foods to your meals, and wean yourself away from the less-healthier ones. (Much more about what to eat coming up in this, and a later chapter.)

Consider the foods and meals and even the snacks you like, and think about the new healthier foods—like vegetables, fruits, fish, whole grains, and low-fat dairy—and then plan your meals around these. Then make a grocery shopping list to help you remember what foods you need.

You may need to watch your budget for food, so shop for healthy options you can afford. Many supermarkets have discount days for seniors; for example, 10% off one day a week, so organize your week so you can stock up on "Senior Day." Check the stores' flyers for other discounts that come up, like lower prices on chicken or low-fat chopped steak, and other sale items. Be sure to sign-up for a free store membership card, which can qualify you for membership-only sales and discounts, like BOGO (buy one; get one).

If you find shopping to be inconvenient or difficult, you now have a multitude of online home delivery shopping options to consider. These range from your local supermarket chain to national chains with healthy food choices like Whole Foods.

There are also online-only services that also let you compose your own shopping list, and deliver to your home. You may see advertising for prepared meals that are home delivered, and promise to help you to lose weight; in checking these out, ensure their recipes contain more natural and less-processed ingredients.

Cooking for 1 or 2

If you were accustomed to cooking for a larger family, you might find it challenging to cook healthy meals for just one or two people. Or you may have lived in a situation where someone else did all the cooking, but now it's up to you.

You may find some days more conducive to meal prep and cooking; it may be due to schedules or appointments, or simply fatigue. Choose to prepare the main meals and snacks on the days when you have the most time and energy. When it's a day when you're too busy or tired to get deeply involved with cooking, select recipes with limited ingredients and require minimal cooking. Or hit the leftovers:

- On those more difficult days, take advantage of what's in the fridge or freezer. "Cook once, eat twice. Make meals that are great as leftovers or make a larger amount and refrigerate or freeze the extras," Canada's *Food Guide* suggests.

Double up by alternating cooking days with the person you live with, or a friend. As well as sharing the work, it creates opportunities to discover one another's recipes and food preferences.

Eating with Others

Eating with other people is great for interacting socially, which has psychological value, and it can also benefit your physical health by encouraging you to eat a diversity of foods that can keep you healthy.

To find ways to share your meals with others, consider joining a lunch club, inviting a neighbor or family member to lunch or dinner at home, and organizing potluck dinners with friends each month, or more often.

Food Guide suggests that you "Check local seniors' community centers and ask about monthly lunches or community kitchens you could join."

Stocking Up

While fresh food is the ideal, having a good stock of non-perishable foods is valuable, and not just for emergencies. Think of the times when you don't have the time or the inclination to shop for today's lunch or tonight's dinner. Maybe it's too hot or too cold; or it's raining or snowing!

On those occasions, it can be a comfort to open the pantry or freezer, and help yourself to the makings of a meal, without stepping outside. Here are some long-lasting foods to stock up on:

- Peanut butter, but go for the all natural versions, with no added salt (or minimal salt), or sugar. Look on-shelf, or grind your own if your market has the set-up. If fresh ground, or once the jar is open, be sure to refrigerate to prevent spoilage. Peanut butter is high in beneficial oils, but be aware of their extra calories.

- Powdered skim milk will keep for months or longer if it stays dry. In addition to making liquid milk, you can add it directly to yogurt, cereals, and a variety of dishes to raise the protein value. Once mixed with water, be sure to refrigerate like regular milk.

    There are storable, long-life alternatives: Sterilized milk, generally packaged in cartons, can last for months, or longer. And you may prefer non-dairy, plant-sourced milk, like soy milk, almond milk, and oat milk. They are high in nutrients, low in fat, but also lower than cow's milk in protein.

- Canned vegetables and fruits have a long shelf life, but be careful to check the label for added salt (listed as sodium) in the vegetables, and added sugar in the fruits. Fortunately, many food producers are responding to the increasing demand to avoid these additives, as well reducing or eliminating preservatives and other chemicals.

- Pasta and its sauces are in a class of their own when it comes to long term storage as well as versatility and simplicity. Pasta sauces can be used at a moment's notice to perk up virtually any meat, fish, or vegetable serving, as well, of course, helping you prepare professional level pasta dishes.

There are endless varieties and brands of pasta sauces in jars and cans; experiment and have fun, but again, check the label for sodium levels. Try whole grain pastas; they may have a stronger flavor that you'll get to like, and the nutritional values are excellent.

- Whole grains like brown rice, quinoa, and oatmeal are easy and fast to prepare, and provide good nutrition. Don't just store them; swap brown rice or quinoa for potatoes on some evenings, and have oatmeal at breakfast, with some raisins, prunes, nuts, seeds, and yogurt mixed in for a powerhouse muesli.

- Protein sources come canned, like the familiar array of fish, including tuna (especially flavorful and nutritious when packed in olive oil; less tasty but lower in calories when water-packed). Same goes for sardines, and mackerel. You can choose from plain, or dressed in sauces. But be wary of canned meats, which can be high in salt and saturated fats.

- Plant-sourced protein-rich canned foods include beans—all types and colors, from black and kidney to lima, pinto and chickpeas (garbanzo), as well as lentils. Canned beans are precooked and just need to be heated before serving, which gives them an advantage over dried beans, which need an overnight soak followed by several hours of simmering!

Freeze it! You can keep a variety of foods in your freezer, including whole grain bread, lean meats, and poultry. Frozen fruits and vegetables are easily defrosted, and tend to be more flavorful and fresher tasting than canned versions.

What to Eat for Protein

Consider this a checklist of 10 foods that should be in a senior's diet, because of their high nutritional values overall, but especially as sources of protein, which is essential for building muscles and strength. We've already covered some of these, but you can use this as a guide for meal planning to be sure you are getting enough protein.

We'll dive deeper into an all-encompassing diet in Chapter 6, and will cover your sources of carbohydrates and fats, but for now, here is the topline on your best sources of protein:

1. **Meat.** Unless you're a vegetarian or vegan, eating lean beef, pork, poultry, and lamb is one of the best ways to get concentrated, nutritionally complete protein: seven grams per ounce, so even a four ounce serving is delivering 28 grams of protein. If chewing is challenging due to gum or dental issues, you can choose ground versions.

2. **Fish.** Cold water, fatty fish, to be specific, like salmon, mackerel, tuna, sardines, and most other ocean-sourced fish. It doesn't matter if the fish is wild-caught or farmed. Fish is equal to meat in supplying complete protein, and its fats are beneficial; low in saturates, and containing antioxidant omega-3 fatty acids.

3. **Eggs.** The once-reviled egg is back with medically-endorsed gusto! Old concerns about cholesterol content have been replaced by recognition of the egg's high quality complete protein, its low level of saturated fats, vitamins, and digestibility. Add to that eggs' good taste however you prepare them, and their low cost relative to other protein sources.

4. **Milk.** Cow's milk, that is. One of nature's most complete foods, milk delivers an impressive eight grams of protein in a glass, along with an array of vitamins (especially D), and minerals (especially calcium for stronger bones). Good carbohydrates too. Most dieticians will encourage fat-free or low fat, but new studies suggest full fat dairy is not bad for you as long as consumed in moderation, albeit there are more calories.

5. **Cheese.** Like milk (from which it is made), cheese is a good source of protein, but many cheeses are high in fat content; you want to go easy on the saturated fats. Softer, fresh cheeses are lower in fat and higher in protein, especially cottage cheese, with its whopping 12 grams of protein in just a half-cup. Cheese can be enjoyed with toast, or sprinkled on a variety of dishes and salads.

6. **Beans.** When beans are served with grains, like rice, pasta, or other whole grains, the already high protein level contributed by the beans is further augmented to achieve nutritionally complete protein; a fact of importance to vegetarians and vegans. As noted in the previous section, be prepared for long soaking and simmering times unless you opt for canned beans. Beans are high in fiber, and help seniors avoid constipation.

7. **Nuts.** Almonds, walnuts, pecans, cashews, macadamias, pistachios, and hazelnuts are excellent sources of monounsaturated oils, protein, and some carbohydrates; they are considered to be one of the healthiest snacks. Just be aware that those healthy oils are high in calories, so don't over do it. Nuts are good additions to salads and cereals.

8. **Peanut Butter.** Surprisingly, peanuts are not really nuts; they're legumes, close to beans, but they have similar protein content to tree nuts. Peanut butter is soft and easy to eat, and can be a good complement to other protein sources. As noted previously, look for all-natural jars, with no added salt or sugar, or grind your own if you are able. Peanut butter is high in beneficial oils, but be aware of their extra calories.

9. **Tofu.** If meat, fish, dairy and eggs are not your thing, you can get nutritionally complete protein from tofu, which is made from soybeans and is relatively inexpensive. Tofu has little taste of its own, but it easily pairs with soups, stews and sauces to absorb their flavor. It's popular in Asian dishes, from cultures where other protein sources were rare. You will find tofu in the refrigerated section of your supermarket or specialty store.

10. **Protein Powders and Shakes.** Most nutritionists and doctors will recommend getting your protein from whole, natural food sources, but if a supplement is needed, for example when there is loss of appetite and reduced consumption, protein powders and shakes can deliver up to 20 grams of protein in a single serving. Look for the least processed, like those based on milk protein.

Anatomy next up. With the fundamentals of nutrition squared away, but just before we get to your ideal diet, the following chapter will give you valuable information about the muscles in your body, and what really happens to those muscles when put to hard work during strength training.

Chapter 5:

Your Anatomy

What Your Muscles Do and How They Work

"Learning basic anatomy for strength training can enhance your results because you will know what and where you are working and identify correctly when you may be compensating," according to physiologist and Master Trainer Elizabeth Leeds, DPT (2015). "Visualization has been shown to increase physical gains, so if you can picture the muscles you are working, you may enhance your results," she adds.

By understanding what your muscles actually are, what they do, and how they communicate with the brain, you will appreciate what your movements, levels of resistance, reps, sets, and rest periods accomplish during your strength training.

Muscle Anatomy

You've seen references to your pecs, quads, lats, abs, glutes, biceps, triceps, and so on, and maybe you recognize the pectorals (pecs) as your chest muscles, the abdominus rectus (abs) as your gut region where you'd like to build a six-pack, or the quadriceps (quads), which are the four big muscles in the front of your thighs.

But now you can learn what each of the major muscle groups are, divided into your upper body, core, and lower body, and showing you their location and function:

Upper Body Muscles

Muscle	Location	Function
Latissimus Dorsi (lats)	Extends up the back and side from pelvis to upper arm.	Enables the arm to reach behind the back.
Pectorals (pecs)	Front of chest, from breastbone to upper arm.	Enables the arm to reach across the chest; helps with lifting.
Anterior Deltoid	Front of upper arm.	Helps raise the arm in front of the body.
Middle Deltoid	Side of upper arm.	Raises the arm upwards and outward to the side.
Posterior Deltoid	Back section of upper arm.	Raises the arm rearward, behind the body.
Biceps	Large muscle in	Enables bending

Muscle	Location	Function
	front of upper arm; runs from shoulder to elbow.	the elbow and helps lift (curl) the arm in front of the body.
Triceps	Primary muscle in back of upper arm; runs from shoulder to elbow.	Enables straightening the elbow and helps lift the arm behind the body.

Mid Body (Core) Muscles

Muscle	Location	Function
Rectus Abdominis (abs)	Lower front section of the trunk; connects lower end of breastbone to pelvis.	Allows the trunk to flex forward and back up.
Obliques	Internal and external obliques extend from lower rib cage to pubic bone.	External obliques rotate trunk to opposite side; internals rotate trunk to same side
Traverse Abdominis	A group of front and back muscles in the lower	Allows compression of lower abdominals

	trunk.	inwards.

Lower Body Muscles

Muscle	Location	Function
Gluteus Maximus (glutes)	Most of the buttock muscle; begins at the pelvis and connects to the upper leg bone (femur).	Extends the leg to the rear. Lower part helps rotate the hip and raise the leg across the body; the upper helps move the leg out to side.
Gluteus Medius	Placed beneath gluteus maximus and connects as well to pelvis and femur.	Helps raise the leg out to the side.
Quadriceps	Composed of four muscle groups in the front of the upper leg; mostly from the pelvis and hip to the knee.	Power standing up, walking, running, jumping. Straightens, raises, and controls the knee.
Hamstrings	The main group of muscles at the rear of the upper leg, connecting the pelvis, hip, and knee.	Allows the knee to bend, and brings the leg to the rear to provide forward propulsion when

Muscle	Location	Function
		walking.
Gastrocnemius (Calves)	The primary muscles at the rear of the lower leg, descending from the knee joint to the Achilles tendon.	Assists with forward walking propulsion, pointing the toes, and raising heels and toes.

Benefits of Exercises to Your Health

We know that exercise, and strength training in particular, benefits virtually every part of your body:

- **Cardio and respiratory.** Exercise strengthens your heart and improves your circulation, helps lower high blood pressure to reduce the risk of strokes, and expands the volume of air and oxygen your lungs can process. The combination of aerobic and resistance training can raise HDL (good) cholesterol and lower LDL (bad) cholesterol. All of these add up to lowering the risk of heart disease.

- **Joints and bones.** Exercise strengthening benefits extend to lubricating your joints, and flexing and strengthening their connective tissues; strengthening your bones by increasing their density, and calming and controlling the digestive system. (More about this under Muscle and Skeletal, below).

- **Disease prevention.** Resistance training helps prevent type 2 diabetes, by inducing reductions in body fat mass, lowering blood pressure, increasing lean muscle body mass, insulin resistance, and glycemic control. There are indications that regular exercise may help prevent many forms of cancer, including "Breast, kidney, colorectal, liver, endometrial, gallbladder, lung, thyroid, ovarian, pancreatic, prostate, gastric, and esophageal" (*Healthline,* 2021). Regular exercise strengthens your immune system, helping to protect you from a wide range of diseases and infections.

- **Weight loss.** Exercise helps keep your weight under control. Dieting alone can slow your metabolism, and make it hard to lose weight. But "Studies have shown that combining aerobic exercise with resistance training can maximize fat loss and muscle mass maintenance," reports *Healthline* (2021), emphasizing the importance of keeping excess weight off while maintaining lean muscle mass.

That's not an all-inclusive list, but it gives you an idea of what's in store for you in response to a serious commitment to resistance training.

But our focus in the chapter is **your muscles,** and there are many muscle-related benefits that will be coming your way:

- **Muscle and skeletal.** Resistance training exercise, first and foremost will build and strengthen your muscles—all of them if you perform full-body routines—which can protect your skeletal structure from injury, while supporting and protecting your joints, especially if they're affected by arthritis.

    "Exercise helps release hormones that promote your muscles' ability to absorb amino acids," *Healthline* explains, which helps your muscles to grow and prevents their breakdown. Resistance training helps prevent sarcopenia, the age-related loss of muscle mass.

- **Coordination.** Strong muscles also improve your stability, coordination and balance, which helps prevent falls, and the injuries they can cause. Strengthening workouts also improve the blood supply to your muscles and their capacity to utilize oxygen more efficiently.

Ergonomics: Psychological and Cognitive

Are you happy? Would you like to become happier, and feel good about yourself? Exercise can elevate your spirit and attitude, and bring feelings of self-confidence and optimism. These are tangible benefits brought on by physical responses to your workouts, including improvements in brain function and cognition:

- Most seniors (and people of all ages) report post-workout improvements in mood, and reductions in anxiety, worry, fear, tension, and depression. These effects are backed up by scientific evidence. *Healthline* reports that exercise has been found to produce "Changes in the parts of the brain that regulate stress and anxiety, and can also increase the brain's sensitivity to the hormones norepinephrine and serotonin, which relieve feelings of depression."

- Exercise also stimulates production of endorphins, which are hormones known to reduce the perception of pain, and produce positive feelings that begin soon after the workout's end, and can last for several hours. It's commonly called the "runner's high," but any good workout seems to create the effect.

- Exercise can improve your brain function, by protecting thinking skills, cognition, and memory.

- When your workout increases your heart rate, it promotes blood and oxygen flow to your brain, while stimulating production of hormones that contribute to the growth of brain cells. Your brain also benefits from exercise's help in preventing chronic diseases.

- Seniors in particular benefit because aging, along with inflammation and oxidative stress can create negative changes in the brain's structure and function. In contrast, brain scans show that exercise is able to cause the hippocampus—the brain's memory and learning center— to increase in size, and potentially improve seniors' mental functioning.

- Exercise is now being credited with slowing or stopping cognitive disorders, including dementia and Alzheimer's.

What else? Exercise that is performed regularly is also helpful in giving you a better night's sleep and overcoming chronic insomnia, improving the health and appearance of your skin, reducing pain perception and increasing pain tolerance, and even improving your sex life. All in all, a good return on your investment of your time and effort exercising.

Your Brain and Muscle Connections

If you're wondering how your muscles know when, and how to move, such as when you go to lift something, or stand, sit, or take a step, here's a summary with the help of Dr. Barbara Kinlay, Ph.D., a professor of psychology at Cornell University who specializes in brain evolution. These neural functions, which are continuous, depend on an amazing system of what we might think of as electrical wiring:

- Muscles only move when they receive commands—signals—from your brain. "Single nerve cells in the spinal cord, called motor neurons, are the only way the brain connects to muscles." So the process begins the moment a motor neuron residing in your spinal cord sends an electrical impulse from your brain to a muscle. The impulse travels along the axon, which is a thin extension of that motor neuron; it's like a tiny bit of voltage going down a very fine wire.

- When the impulse has traversed the length of the axon to reach the muscle, it causes a chemical reaction that stimulates the muscle. It helps to know that muscles are built of long fibers connected to each lengthwise, "By a ratchet mechanism that allows two parts of an extension ladder to slide past each other and then lock in a certain position."

- So the instant the impulse from the motor neuron reaches the muscle, it causes "Muscle fibers to ratchet past each other and overlap, so that the muscle gets shorter and fatter." This is a muscle contraction, which continues until the motor neuron impulses stop, allowing the muscle fibers to slide back to their original positions, and relax the contraction.

Okay, but how does the message to lift, stand, or step originate, before it heads down the axon as an impulse to the muscle? It's a multi-stage process that begins in your brain's cerebral cortex, where a series of commands develop among the neurons responsible for coordinated movements:

- "In your brain the cerebral cortex connects to a sort of console in the spinal cord that overlays the motor neurons." This console specifies the positions of arms and legs, for example, including the directions of expected movements. This quickly evolves into a collection of specific commands to each motor neuron and muscle.

- "Each motor neuron connects to just one muscle, like the bicep on the front of your upper arm that lifts your forearm, or to the triceps, on the back of your upper arm that extends your forearm" (Finlay, 2015).

Joints and Pain

If you think that joint aches and pains are part of the aging process, you won't be surprised to learn that 50% of adults over the age of 65 are experiencing at least some degree of joint pain (*WebMD*, 2021).

But joint pain does not have to be inevitable; healthy lifestyle changes, including strengthening exercises, can reduce or prevent joint-related injuries and conditions. "Pain is more common as we age, but not necessarily a fact of life," according to Rhett Smith, DO, a rheumatologist (Smith, 2021).

Types of Joint Pain and its Causes

There are many causes of joint pain among seniors, ranging from years of use and activity to injuries and autoimmune reactions, but regardless of the origins, most joint pains trace to two conditions:

- **Osteoarthritis** (OA) is the more common type of arthritis, and it affects 27 million Americans, especially seniors. "Osteoarthritis is often called wear and tear arthritis because it comes from using your joints over time or after an injury" (*WebMD,* 2021). It's caused principally when the "Cartilage that cushions the ends of the bones in your joints wears away," and when that happens, the bones that form the joints rub against each other, creating friction, and pain.

- **Rheumatoid** arthritis (RA) is a chronic inflammatory condition caused by the immune system attacking the tissues that lines the joints. Symptoms, in addition to pain, may include swollen joints, tenderness, stiffness, as well as fatigue, loss of appetite, and fever.

Lifestyle changes may be helpful in preventing or relieving OA. It's best to start with recognizing which joints are most susceptible to overuse or improper use trauma, and the longer term damage and pain that results.

"High-traffic joints like knees, lower back, neck, shoulders, toes, and the base of the thumb are likely spots for OA joint pain due to injuries and extra weight" when the person is overweight or obese (*WebMD,* 2021). Arthritis frequently affects the hands because of injuries, or heavy use; there may be a genetic predisposition.

Preventing Joint Pain

Here are lifestyle or behavioral changes that can reduce trauma and injury to your joint, and prevent the onset of pain, or reduce the discomfort if pain is already present. You'll find that most of these modifications have other important health benefits, from heart and lung health to cancer prevention:

Stop smoking. On top of not smoking to avoid cardiovascular and respiratory damage, and the risks of cancer, smokers should consider the negative effects of smoking on the immune system, which can make you more susceptible to RA. Smoking also increases sensitivity to the pain of OA, and can reduce the effectiveness of certain medications. If you are a smoker and find it hard to quit, check out support groups.

Lose extra weight. If you are overweight, or especially if obese, losing weight can take a lot of pressure off the joints, especially the hips, knees, and ankles. *WebMD* cites a study that shows that losing even one pound can take up to four pounds of pressure off of the knee joints, so a loss of 10 lbs can translate to 40 lbs less of a load for the knees to support. Your heart will thank you for heading toward a normal weight too.

Be active. Avoid being sedentary, and keep moving; this is another lifestyle change that has lots of benefits. Your joints will appreciate resistance exercises, which will strengthen their supportive muscles. Just be sure to never put your joints under too much pressure; if the activity hurts, stop.

But consider the types of your workouts to determine where you might be able to reduce the stress; for example, no longer jogging on a hard surface, which can lead to runner's knee— when the kneecap cartilage abrades, letting the joint components rub roughly against each other. Instead get your aerobic conditioning on a treadmill, stair-climber, or elliptical. Or by walking, swimming laps, or cycling.

Posture. Standing and walking upright distributes your weight evenly over your hip joints and knees, and keeps your spinal column aligned to protect the vertebrae from damage or wear. Good posture will help prevent bending forward of your neck and thoracic spine (kyphosis), and make you less susceptible to falling.

How to ensure good posture? Consider this advice from West Hartford Health & Rehab Center (WHHR) (2020): "A strong core makes it easier to maintain proper posture, reducing stress on your spinal and cervical joints."

Eat healthy. We keep coming back to the importance of a good diet for all aspects of your health, including keeping your joints strong and flexible; we'll delve deeper into diet in the next chapter. "A healthy diet includes fresh fruits and vegetables and cooking from scratch to avoid processed foods," according to Elena Schiopu, MD, who is a professor of rheumatology at the University of Michigan (*WebMD*). "It's time consuming, but we must invest in our health, including our joint health, which will determine our quality of life as we get older."

Avoid sugar is an especially concerning food to watch out for; it's loading beverages, cereals, pastries and baked goods with "empty calories," meaning they bring no nutritional value, while contributing to weight gain, and causing insulin-challenging spikes to glucose in the blood. Sugar consumption can cause chronic inflammation, triggering autoimmune attacks on the joints, leading to RA-induced swelling and pain.

So steer clear of sugary soft drinks, fruit juices with added sugar, and even sports beverages that contain sugar. Choose water to stay well hydrated to keep your joints lubricated.

Sleep well. Forget the high-powered types who brag about only needing a few hours sleep; we all need at least seven to eight hours of sleep every night, so our brains can recharge, and our bodies can rebuild. Lack of sleep can lead to increased joint pain, as well as depression.

Go to sleep and wake up at the same time every night, including weekends, so your body gets used to the pattern. Don't have coffee or black tea for hours before bedtime (some caffeine-free alternatives may be okay). Be careful too with alcohol before retiring; it may actually awaken you after an hour or two. Put down digital devices at least an hour before bed, since their screens can be stimulating. Some seniors find that light yoga stretching or meditation can relax and help them fall asleep.

Physical therapy. A lack of mobility caused by joint degeneration and its pain can make things worse. WHHR encourages movement, advising "Physical therapy can get these joints moving, without additional stress or accelerating damage." Those who achieve a "Greater range of motion may find they're able to participate in low-impact activities that may have been difficult before."

Plan your diet! Now that you have a better understanding of what your muscles are, what they do, and how they communicate with your brain, as well as knowing about your joints, and how to protect them, you are ready to advance to nutritional training as the next phase of your strength training.

Chapter 6:

Your Diet Plan

Add Life to Your Years; Add Years to Your Life

With the basics and principles of nutrition already covered, this chapter will give you a good start in learning how to adopt, enjoy, and benefit from a highly nutritious diet. Here you will find examples of simple diet plans, ranging from the regular to the Mediterranean.

It includes some tips on how to keep up and stay with a successful diet by making it part of your overall lifestyle, and especially your successful strength training journey.

What is a successful diet? Think beyond just calories or building muscle mass; think of taking nutrition and your health seriously, even if it means modifying eating habits and ways of thinking of food. A good, healthy diet can protect you from diseases and conditions that can diminish your well-being and even shorten your life, so enter into this as an adventure into diet along with exercise that will add to your health, satisfaction, and strength.

Tips for a Healthy Diet

Loving what you eat will come easily when your meals and snacks not only taste great, but are great for you. It's a win-win situation! These tips will get you started on the right track to nutritional triumph:

Advance Meal Planning. It makes sense to think and plan, rather than leaving your meals to a last minute scramble for ingredients, and often realizing you haven't allowed enough time for preparation and cooking.

- Planning will keep you organized. "Meal planning takes the guesswork out of eating and can help ensure you eat a variety of nutritious foods throughout the day" (National Institute on Aging [NIA], 2022).

- Prepping and cooking can (and should) be a relaxing, creative experience, and it can be, if you plan. There's no reason to turn these activities into stressful, rushed, and frustrating scenarios, which can happen without planning.

- A good way to become an effective planner is to pick a time each week, like Sunday afternoons, when you will remember to devote a few minutes to planning both the week's meals and your workouts. This will take the guesswork out of "What's for dinner tonight?" and digging around the fridge and freezer for "potluck."

- Planning your meals and menus will ensure that you are eating the foods you should be eating, regularly. Don't worry if you aren't able to plan every lunch and dinner; plan what you can at first, and in time you'll have a large repertory of familiar and favorite meals to put into the planner.

Write it down. This will give you a roadmap to guide your shopping selections, and can prove you with a shopping list. A market usually has a dazzling array of selections in every category of foods, from fruits and vegetables to meats and fish. A list can keep you focused and not be overwhelmed by the variety.

- But be open to new ideas and options that you discover while shopping, especially if certain items of interest are on sale or offered as BOGO (Buy One; Get One). Be flexible; there's no reason you can't make substitutions when something appeals to your appetite or your budget!

- Good professional chefs and serious cooks let the freshness and quality of the market's offerings influence their selections of ingredients.

Preparation time. Unless you are an experienced cook, you may be surprised how much time can go into preparation and cooking. There may be peeling, chopping, sauteing, and even pre-soaking, and marinating that can require an earlier start to the meal prep.

- Be especially conscious of time requirements when serving others, and it's not just you at lunch or dinner; you don't want to keep your hungry guests waiting.

- A tip is to prepare meals in advance that don't need your attention in the half-hour or hour before serving; stews, hearty soups, and casserole dishes, for example (or anything that simmers or cooks all day, if you have a slow-cooking machine).

- Another heads up for when others are involved: Don't get yourself tied up in the kitchen when you'd rather be socializing. If you keep the meal simple—think of cooking everything in one pot—you'll free up prep time, and have less to clean up afterward.

Manage calories. You do not have to become obsessed with counting every calorie you consume, but it's important to manage your intake, which can be done by observing certain guidelines.

- First, limit how much you eat, and try to cut back on large quantities, big servings, and second helpings. A good way to do this without feeling hungry is to start your meal with a low calorie, yet filling, bowl of soup or a salad (but with minimal dressing). This is known as volumetrics, and it's a good way to get valuable nutrients too.

- The second broad guideline is to avoid foods that are high in hidden calories, or at least consume them with moderation. We all love apple pie (or cherry, or blueberry), but check the calories and you will be amazed: There's lots of sugar in the pie filling, and more in the crust, where you will also find quite a bit of high-calorie hydrogenated fat from shortening.

Beware of sugar. But let's get back to sugar. The problem with sugar, which is a molecule called sucrose, is that it contains calories, four per gram like all carbohydrates, but without any nutritional value, and unlike carrots or oatmeal, it's easy to eat too much sugar. Natural or unrefined sugar, and maple and agave syrups are pretty close to refined sugar. Honey too, except that the bees have partially predigested it.

- All sugars have a high glycemic index, meaning they send too much glucose into the blood, which is a real issue for diabetics, and to a lesser degree, for all of us due to the need for insulin reaction to moderate the glucose.

- As mentioned previously, sugar can be found in soft drinks, snacks and pastries, sports beverages, and most breakfast cereals, especially the presweetened varieties. Choose a nutritious alternative: Give highly high fiber oatmeal a try, and toss in some fruit (fresh or dry), and some nuts or seeds.

- Check the labels on your favorite ice cream, and note the amounts of saturated fat and carbs from, you guessed it, sugar. And yes, the ice cream calories count even when you eat directly from the container! You may be surprised to know that the most expensive brands of ice cream tend to be highest in sugar and fat, and of course, calories. Yogurt is a great, healthy alternative, but when fresh or frozen, heads up on the sugar content. It's best to go with sugar-free yogurt, with added fruit for sweetness and flavor.

Know your nutrients. Almost every food that is packaged has a Nutrition Facts panel, which lets you see at a glance the per serving calories, carbs, saturated and total fats, and protein, as well as sodium, fiber, vitamins and minerals. As you shop, let these panels inform your purchase decisions.

- As *Vantage Aging* (2021) advises, "Nutrients in foods help our bodies stay healthy and active. Knowing which nutrients are important will help you decide what kinds of foods to eat." Healthy meals should include a "Variety of brightly colored foods," especially vegetables and fruits, whole grains, beans, nuts and seeds, and protein from lean meats, fish (fresh and canned), low-fat dairy, and eggs.

- "Look for foods that are high in fiber and Vitamin D. Avoid foods with high salt (sodium) content, and avoid canned processed, preserved meats.

The Mediterranean Diet

We've mentioned it before; now let's take a deeper dive into what many medical and nutritional authorities believe to be the ideal healthy diet for almost everyone. Unlike many of the popular fad diets, with the Mediterranean diet there is no overloading on fats or protein, no avoidance of carbohydrates, no skipping meals, and no fasting. Instead of the demands of many poorly researched diets, there are no gimmicks or sacrifices that have to be made.

This diet that has evolved over the generations has proven to be heart healthy, as well as reducing the risks of many other diseases, and providing energy, endurance, and strength.

The keywords here are balanced, natural, unprocessed, and lifestyle, because those who live in the Mediterranean Basin, and whose diet this is based upon, also keep physically active, know how to stay calm and stress-free, and are interactive socially. This diet helps them to manage their weight without starving themselves. It is the combination of all of these factors that contribute to their health, happiness, and longevity.

Just before we get into the practical realities of the diet, here is a reprise of the food groups that are its components:

- **Vegetables** of every kind and color. Green lettuces, kale, peppers, spinach, broccoli, brussels sprouts, celery, cucumbers, peas, string beans, and asparagus; yellow squash, peppers, corn; red tomatoes, peppers, beets; plus carrots, potatoes, sweet potatoes, avocados, onions, shallots, leeks, and various other types according to seasonal availability.

- **Fruits,** including fresh apples, pears, melons, grapes, peaches, nectarines, oranges and tangerines, kiwis, bananas, pineapples, mangos, and papayas. Plus dried apricots, prunes, dates, and raisins (but note the high calories in dried fruits).

- **Whole grains,** like oats, whole wheat and rye, quinoa, barley, farro, and brown rice. Use directly, or in breads, cereals and muesli, and pasta. You'll quickly discover the richer flavor of whole grains, along with benefiting from their nutrients and fiber. Read the labels; multigrain does not mean whole grain!

- **Nuts,** including walnuts, pecans, cashews, macadamia, pistachios, and hazelnuts. **Seeds,** like flax, chia, pumpkin, and sunflower.

- **Beans,** of every color, from red kidney and pinto to black, white, and lima. Lentils and chickpeas belong here; so do peanuts, since they resemble beans biologically, and grow underground, not on trees. These foods are called legumes.

- **Lean meats,** with no visible fat, and served in small quantities (a deck of cards size): beef, lamb, veal, pork, chicken and turkey.

- **Fish,** ideally cold-water sourced, like salmon, tuna, mackerel, cod, haddock, halibut, and sardines; all these have beneficial fats including Omega-3 fatty acids.

- **Dairy,** primarily low-fat and non-fat: milk, yogurt, cottage cheese, and aged cheeses, but in moderation, given their high saturated fat content.

- **Eggs** have regained their positive image as a healthy source of protein, vitamins, and minerals. One egg a day is the recommended serving.

- **Olive oil** (extra virgin, which is cold pressed and minimally processed) and avocado oil are considered the best for health given their high levels of monounsaturated fats.

How To: Mediterranean Diet in Action

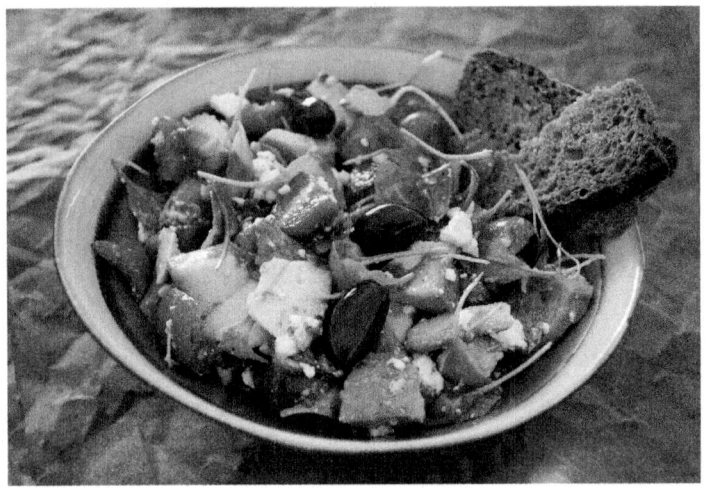

Now that you are aware of what the Mediterranean diet contains, here are the practical actions you should take to make this diet *your diet,* what you can call your Mediterranean diet "do" list:

- Make olive oil your go-to, regular oil, and use it exclusively in cooking, and for seasoning dishes.

- Eat at least two or three servings of cooked vegetables daily, and, at least one serving of fresh vegetables in a salad, or as crudités (sliced, chunked).

- Have a minimum of two or three servings of fresh fruit daily; have dried fruits on occasion.

- Eat at least three servings of beans (legumes) every week.

- Have three servings of fish or other types of seafood each week, make at least one serving (ideally two) be fatty cold-water fish.

- At least one serving of nuts or seeds each week; this is a minimum, and your regular, frequent consumption ,especially of seeds, is encouraged.

- White meat from chicken and turkey should replace red meat twice a week, or avoid having any meat a few days a week. Try to avoid processed meats in sausages, bacon, and salami.

- Create a customized sauce of tomato, onion or shallots, and (optionally) garlic, by simmering these in olive oil. Add your favorite herbs, but go easy on the salt. Use to dress vegetables, pasta dishes, rice and other grains, and even eggs, fish and seafood.

- If you drink alcoholic beverages, let wine (especially red) be your preferred form, but limit consumption to one or two glasses per day.

- For desserts, choose fruits instead of sugary pastries and ice cream (or at least minimize their consumption. Enjoy dark chocolate—at least 70% cacao, which is high in antioxidants, and very low in sugar.

- Lower stress by not always eating "on the run." Have at least two meals every day being seated at the table for 20 minutes or longer. Slow down your eating by not taking a spoonful or forkful until you swallow the previous bite. Become aware of your chewing and swallowing to become mindful.

Now that you know what the Mediterranean diet consists of, and how it can be put into action, let's consider what this diet keeps you away from; a "don'ts" list:

- Cream and butter, which are very high in fat overall, and saturated fats in particular. Margarine and shortening may be free of animal fats, but are hydrogenated to make them solid, and end up equally high in saturated fats and calories.

- Cold cuts or delicatessen meats, like salami, bologna, liverwurst. Also preserved and canned meats, like pâté, Spam. Watch out too for sausages, and most forms of bacon. Same goes for cured ham.

- Refined grains that have been stripped of their outer, nutrient-rich coatings, like white flour that's used in white breads, and even "rye" and "multi-grain," and cereals and pastas. Check the labels.

- Soft drinks, whether carbonated or not, and all other sweetened beverages, including sports replenishment drinks, and any fruit juices that have sugar added.

- Pies, cakes, and other pastries, doughnuts (which are fried in oil), puddings, cookies, and custards, especially if commercially produced. Ice cream varies in fat and sugar levels; read the labels, and eat ice cream, gelato, and even sweetened yogurt with restraint, or rarely.

- French fries and potato chips, which are deep fried in oils that may contain trans fats and toxins, and add loads of fat calories to previously low fat, nutritious potatoes. Popcorn is a natural, fat-free alternative (as long as you don't load it up with butter and salt!).

The list of "don'ts" is not an ironclad "thou shalt not" dictum without flexibility. You don't have to give up bacon, doughnuts, fries, or ice cream for the rest of your life. But recognize the dangers these foods can pose to your health, and muscle building, and wean them out of your diet as much as you can. You do not want to negate the good "dos" of the Mediterranean diet.

Mediterranean Daily Menu Planning

You are free, of course, to select any variety of foods to create your own Mediterranean diet, but with the help of nutrition expert Jon Johnson in *Medical News Today* (2022), here are a few day's menus to get your inspiration started:

Day 1

Breakfast

- One egg, scrambled or pan-fried in a thin film of butter (yes, butter is okay and good for you if used sparingly).

- Whole grain toast, topped with a couple of slices of grilled tomatoes. For a more filling breakfast, make it two eggs, or add a few slices of avocado to the toast.

Lunch

- Mixed salad greens (about two cups) with cherry or chopped tomatoes, celery, sliced mushrooms, and olives, and with a dressing of extra virgin olive oil and apple cider vinegar. For extra calories and to make it more filling, top with canned tuna in olive oil, or a few bites of meat.

- Whole grain pita bread, or whole grain toasted bread, with two oz hummus spread.

Dinner

- Pizza made with whole grain crust, and tomato sauce, and topped with grilled vegetables, and low-fat cheese, like mozzarella, or a mixture of low-fat cheeses if not sure about fat levels, use sparingly.

- To make it a hardier meal, add tuna, pine nuts, or shredded chicken. Any mushrooms or olives left over from lunch can be added too.

Day 2

Breakfast

- One cup of Greek or Icelandic-style yogurt (highest in protein). Choose fat-free or low-fat versions.

- Half cup of fruits, such as raspberries, blueberries, chopped peaches or nectarines. Add a tablespoon or walnuts, pecans, almonds, or cashew for extra calories and more nutrients. You can mix the fruit with the yogurt, or eat separately.

- One slice of toasted whole grain bread, lightly buttered (it's okay; see Day 1).

Lunch

- A whole grain sandwich filled with grilled vegetables, like zucchini and eggplant, plus onion and green or red bell pepper. To add some extra calories, nutrition, and flavor, spread some avocado or hummus on the bread.

Dinner

- Baked salmon, halibut, or cod with chopped shallots and ground pepper for extra flavor. Try coating the fish with some balsamic vinegar before baking for a sweet and tangy marinated effect.

- Roasted potato with extra virgin olive oil and fresh, chopped herbs, like dill or chives.

Day 3

Breakfast

- A cup of cooked whole grain oatmeal (made from a half cup of dry oats and low-fat milk or water), with cinnamon, chopped dates, and a teaspoon of honey; optional, for added sweetness.

- Top with raspberries, blueberries, or blackberries (or sliced strawberries), or any chopped fruit. Add the fruit after cooking the oatmeal. Optional: Add a spoonful of sliced almonds or other nuts, either before or after cooking, as you prefer; the cooked nuts will be soft, but if uncooked, they'll be crunchy.

Lunch

- White beans (or any color or type you prefer, like black, kidney, chickpeas or lima) with herbs, like cumin, oregano, thyme, laurel, or basil (fresh, if available). About a half cup serving of beans is about right; they're high in protein and calories so they tend to be satiating (filling). You can use lentils instead of beans.

- A cup (or more, if you love salads) of arugula with an extra virgin olive oil dressing, and topped with chunks or slices of tomatoes, cucumbers, and Greek feta cheese, which is low-fat.

Dinner

- A half cup of cooked whole grain pasta (any shape), topped with tomato sauce (homemade, ideally), extra virgin olive oil, and grilled vegetables. Add pieces of leftover chicken to increase the protein and make the dish more filling.

- Sprinkle a tablespoon of grated Parmesan cheese on top for added flavor and nutrients, but not too many calories.

NIA Daily Menu Planning

The National Institute on Aging (NIA) has published lists of daily menus that are based on values similar to the Mediterranean diet that you can also refer to. Detailed recipes can easily be found on line; for example, turkey tetrazzini or quesadillas:

Breakfast

- Yogurt smoothie with fruit and spinach.

- Vegetable omelet served on or with whole grain toast.

- Avocado slices with bruschetta.

- Oatmeal or muesli with banana.

- Eggs over sweet potato grits (or corn grits) and spinach or kale.

Lunch

- Chicken sandwich on whole grain bread, with sliced avocado and tomato.

- Quinoa stir-fried with mixed chopped vegetables.

- Apple coleslaw as a side dish.

- Sweet potato quesadillas with black beans.

- Sanchico tuna salad with chopped tomatoes, avocado, onion, and red peppers.

Dinner

- Chicken breast roasted with vegetables and hummus.

- Roasted or broiled salmon, with roasted sweet potato and zucchini.

- Whole wheat pasta, mixed with ground turkey, shallots, and tomato sauce.

- Grilled sirloin steak (or other very lean cut), lightly salted.

- Turkey tetrazzini, with whole wheat pasta, peas, and broth.

- Steamed fish with broccoli, kale, or spinach.

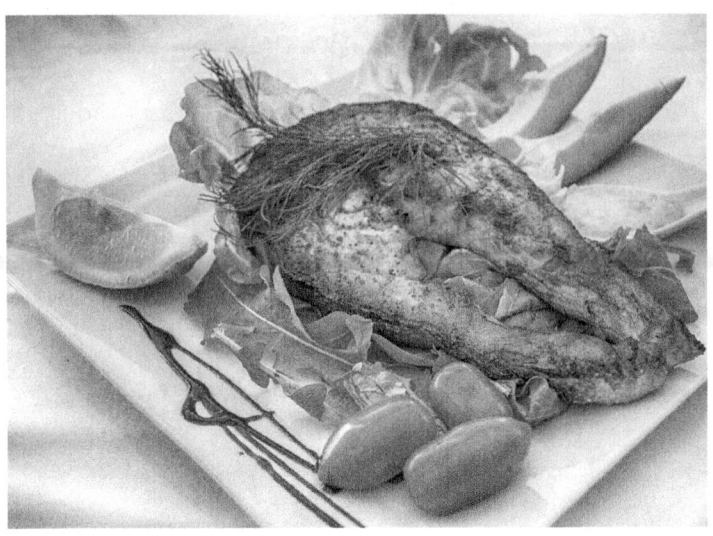

Healthy Snacks

- Baby carrots or carrot sticks with hummus dip.
- Celery sticks filled with natural peanut butter.
- Greek or Icelandic yogurt with fruit.
- Banana, cocoa, and yogurt pops, mixed and frozen.
- Popcorn flavored with butter (small amount) and chili powder.
- Bean dip with yogurt and salsa, well mixed.

As we conclude this chapter, it's important to recognize the close relationship between nutrition and exercise in building strength and muscle mass. Your body needs the right nutrients, including more protein than normal to repair and rebuild muscle tissue.

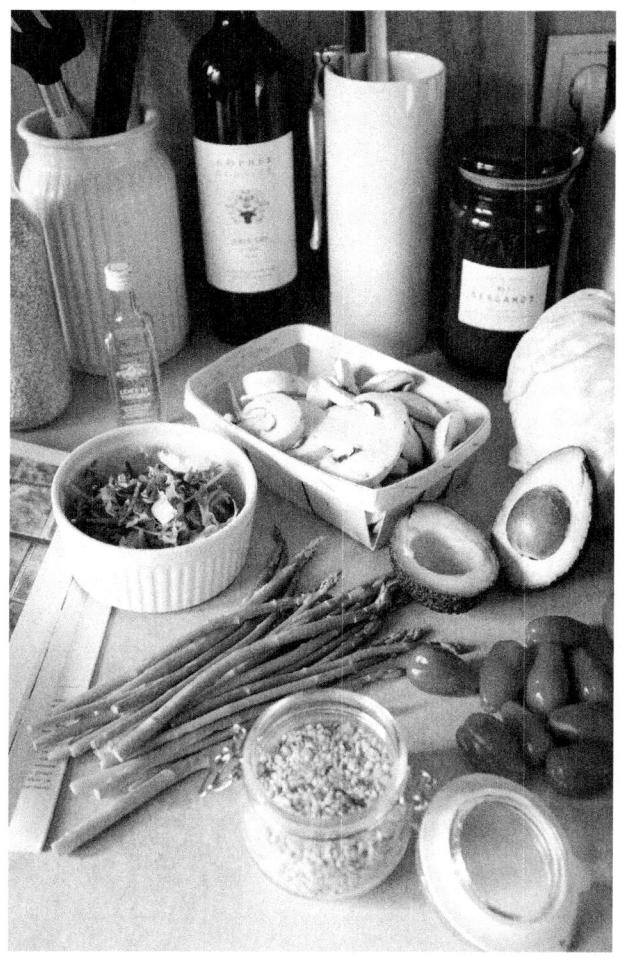

You are ready now to start the strength training instructions. We'll begin with the basic exercises, before moving on to more complex routines.

Chapter 7:

The Basic Exercises

You Can Start at Home Today

The best way for you to begin your strengthening exercises is to get started now, rather than later; don't put off your training until you've acquired equipment, or join a fitness center. Starting now means today, or tomorrow, while your interest and enthusiasm is high, and you're anxious to begin getting stronger. The sooner you begin, the sooner you'll be able to see and feel your progress!

To ensure you can get going now, we'll concentrate on simple exercises—the basics that you can easily learn, and do at home. These basic exercises can be incorporated into your 10 week program, and from squats and push ups to toe raises, these simple at home exercises can go a long way to help you to regain your strength.

Just remember to take things slowly, and learn how to do them right for optimal results, as well as for safety.

Basic Bodyweight Exercises

Squats to Chair

Squats strengthen the lower body, especially the quads, and the midbody core to help you to stand up, walk, climb stairs, and bend to lift objects.

- **How to:** Stand in front of a chair with feet hip-width apart. Hold your chest upright as you shift your hips back and bend at the knees to lower your bottom toward the chair.

  Just touch the chair or sit on it, as you pause, then press down with your feet and legs to rise, slightly leaning forward and tightening your glutes as you return to standing. Protect your knees by keeping your weight mostly over your heels and feet.

- **How many:** Perform 3 sets of 10 reps, with 60 seconds rest between sets.

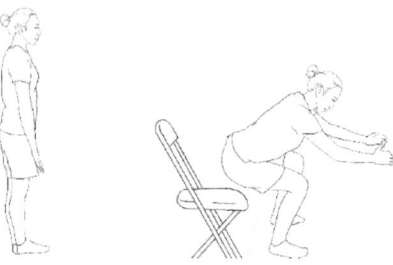

Wall Push Ups

Your arms, shoulders, chest, upper back and core benefit from this modified push up. Your entire upper body and abs will strengthen.

- **How to:** Stand facing a wall, with toes about 2 feet away from the wall, extend your arms fully and place your hands on it at shoulder height and width apart. Keep your body in a straight line as you bend at the elbows to lower your head and chest to the wall. Try to keep your heels on the floor. Pause, then slowly push with your hands to straighten your arms and return to starting position. Tip: If you find this too difficult, stand closer to the wall.

- **How many:** Perform 3 sets of 12 to 14 reps, with 45 to 60 seconds rest between sets.

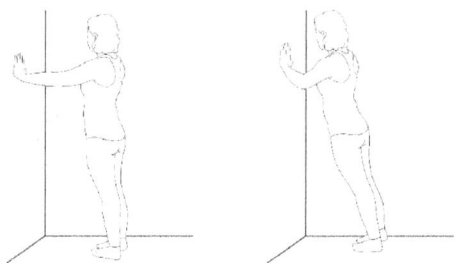

Quadruped Opposite Arm and Leg Balance

This exercise helps improve your coordination, balance, and strength in the abs and back muscles.

- **How to:** Get down on all fours with hands beneath your shoulders and knees below your hips. Keep your abdominals tight and back flat as you raise one arm to extend directly in front of your shoulder, and raise and extend your opposite leg directly behind your hip. Hold for up to three exhales, then lower your arm and leg, and repeat on the opposite side.

- **How many:** Perform 3 sets of 6 to 8 reps, with 45 seconds rest between sets.

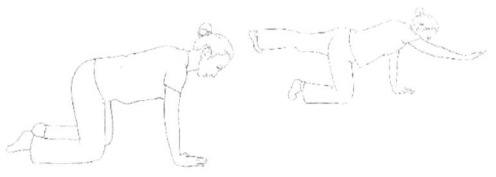

Wall Angels

This will open your chest to improve your posture and ease lower back tightness and pain, and increase shoulder range of motion.

- **How to:** Stand with your back against a wall, and the back of your head touching the wall, and with your feet about 6 inches out from the wall. Hold your arms down by your sides, and tuck your chin toward your chest. Turn your palms facing forward and slowly swing your arms outward, keeping them straight and in contact with the wall.

    Keep raising your arms without bending your elbows and reaching for the ceiling (if you can). Pause, then lower your straight, unbent arms to your sides, keeping wall contact.

- **How many:** Perform 3 sets of 8 to 10 reps, with 30 to 45 seconds rest between sets.

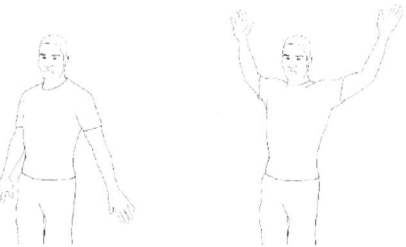

Wall Slides

Your posture will improve and your lower joints will be less painful as you strengthen your hip flexors and knees with these slides; a variation of squats.

- **How to:** Stand and lean your upper and lower back, shoulders, arms and head against a wall, placing your feet about 1 to 2 feet forward. Bend your knees to squat, lowering your body to nearly 90 degrees. Pause in the position for three exhales, and slide back up.

- **How many:** Perform 2 sets of 10 reps, with 45 to 60 seconds rest between sets.

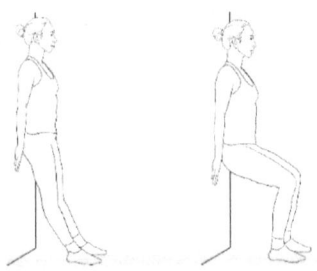

Pec Stretches

Your posture will improve as you stretch and loosen tight pecs in your chest. It will loosen your shoulders too.

- **How to:** Stand in a doorway and place your hands on the sides, at about head height. Step into the doorway with either foot and lean forward, feeling the opening of your chest. Hold the position for 20 seconds. Tip: Vary the height of your hands to extend the stretch.

- **How many:** Perform 3 20-second stretches, with 30 seconds rests.

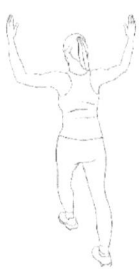

Standing Balance

This will help improve your balance; over time, you will be able to perform this movement for longer intervals.

- **How to:** Stand facing a counter, desk, table, or the back of a chair, and place one or both hands lightly on top for steadiness. Without leaning, lift one foot off the floor and hold this position as long as you can. Lower your foot, and lift your other foot, and keep it up for 20 seconds, or as long as you can.

- **How many:** Perform 1 or 2 reps. With practice, you should be able to keep each foot up for a full minute, without holding on.

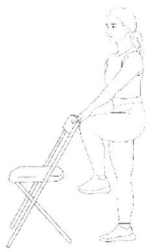

Chin Up

This is more of a practice than an exercise; it will help relieve neck pain and improve your posture.

- **How to:** Become aware of your head's position as you stand and walk, and avoid letting your head bend forward. Keep your neck and head upright, in alignment with your hips. This will take pressure off your neck, upper spine (thoracic), and shoulders.

- **How many:** Make checking your posture a habit. Be aware as you sit, too.

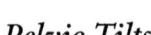

Pelvic Tilts

You will stretch and strengthen your lower back with this subtle movement of your hips and contraction of your glutes.

- **How to:** Pelvic tilts may be performed lying on your back or while standing. Tighten your buttocks and roll your hips forward. Hold for 3 seconds, then roll your hips back and relax your buttocks. Unlike other exercises, there is not much movement, but with practice you will feel the benefits.

- **How many:** Do 8 to 12 reps, once or twice every day.

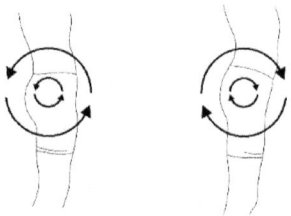

Shoulder Blade Squeezes

Your chest muscles (pecs) will open, allowing your posture to improve. There will also be some increased range of motion in your shoulders.

- **How to:** Stand upright, with good posture, and with hands at your sides. Pull your shoulders back, and try to bring your shoulder blades together (they won't touch, but it's the effort that counts). Keep your shoulders down, not hunched. You can extend the stretch by bending your arms and pulling your elbows rearward and toward each other.

- **How many:** Hold the squeeze for 3 to 5 seconds, then release. Do 8 to 12 reps.

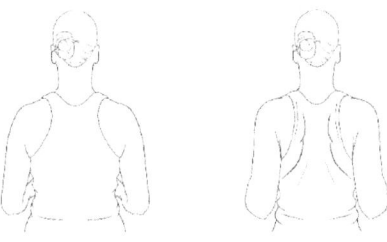

Toe Taps

Your lower legs—both calves and shins—will strengthen and blood circulation will be improved with these simple toe lifts.

- **How to:** Sit in a chair and have both feet flat, pointed ahead. Keeping the heels down, raise your toes, as if trying to touch your shins, then lower to the floor, in one continuous motion.

- **How many:** Do 20 to 30 reps, once or twice every day.

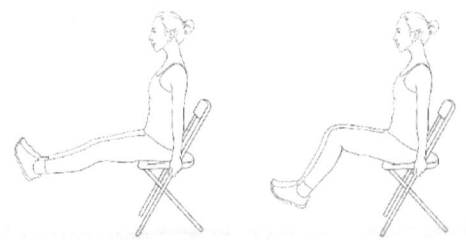

Heel Raises

The calves benefit from this similar exercise to toe taps.

- **How to:** Sit and have both feet flat, pointed ahead. Keeping the toes down, raise your heels as if trying to touch your calves, then lower to the floor, in one continuous motion.

- **How many:** Do 20 to 30 reps, once or twice every day.

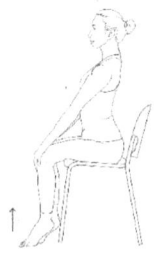

Knee Lifts

The quad muscles in your thighs will be strengthened, and the hips and glutes will be flexed.

- **How to:** Sit with feet close together, and raise your right knee so your right foot is about 6 inches off the floor. Hold for 3 seconds, then lower to complete one movement. You may continue the reps with the right leg, then switch to the left leg; or alternate with each leg for each lift.

- **How many:** A total of 10 to 14 lifts with each leg, rest, then repeat one more set.

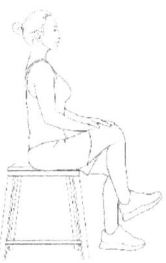

Toe Stands

If walking has become more difficult due to stiffening of joints and lower muscle strength, these toe stands will strengthen calves and ankles, and improve stability and balance.

- **How to:** Stand facing a counter or table, or the back of a chair, and rest your fingers on it for balance (but don't lean on it). Rise up on the balls of your feet and toes as high as you can, and hold for 3 to 4 seconds, then lower back down. Pause for 4 seconds, then repeat.

  Tip: For more intensity, stand on a step with the front of your feet, so your heels can go lower when you come back down.

- **How many:** Do 10 reps, then rest for 60 seconds and do another set of 10.

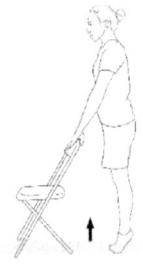

Finger Marching

You will engage your fingers, hands, and arms, resulting in strengthening your grip and upper body, and flexing your arms, shoulders, and back.

- **How to:** Stand, or sit on the forward part of a chair, with your feet shoulder-width apart. Raise your arms toward the ceiling, and wiggle your fingers for 10 seconds, then lower your arms.

  Next, reach behind your back, trying to reach your elbows; hold for 10 seconds then relax. Finally, interlace your fingers and extend your arms outward, parallel to the floor, and pull so your shoulders roll forward. Hold for 10 seconds.

- **How many:** Repeat the 3 movements 3 times. Pause to rest as needed.

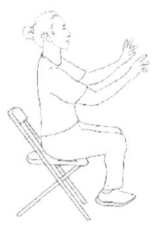 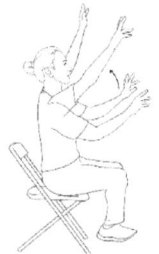

Step-Ups

Your hips, upper and lower legs, ankles, and buttocks will strengthen, and your balance will improve with these simple step-ups.

- **How to:** Stand at the bottom of a staircase; you may lightly hold on to the railing, if needed for balance. Step up with your left leg and place your foot onto the first step. Now step up with the right foot, and place it next to the left foot.

  Pause for a moment, then lower your right foot back down; this is one rep. After completing the desired reps, reverse the exercise with the right foot on the step, and the left foot going up and down.

- **How many:** Repeat 10 times with each leg for 1 set. Rest for 40 seconds and do a second set.

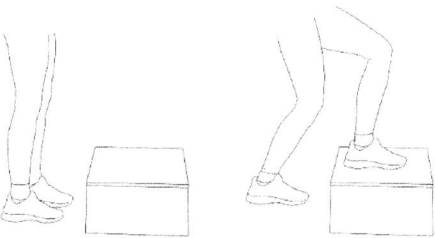

Side Hip Raise

Targets your hips, thighs, and buttocks muscles to shape and firm your lower body, and helps protect your hips from fractures.

105

- **How to:** Stand behind a sturdy chair or table, and steady yourself by placing your hands on it. Your feet should be slightly apart; toes pointing forward. Raise your left leg out to the side; move slowly, and don't lock your knees. You do not have to raise the leg too high. Pause, then slowly lower the leg down. Repeat with your right leg. This is 1 rep.

- **How many:** Repeat 10 times with each leg for 1 set. Rest for 30 to 40 seconds, and do a second set.

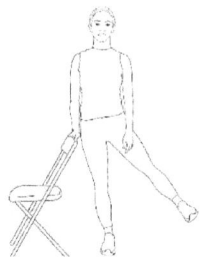

Knee Extension

You can strengthen weak and arthritic knees by building the quad muscles that support the knees.

- **How to:** You'll need ankle weights to increase resistance. Sit well back in a chair with both feet pointed forward. Slowly raise one leg to horizontal (or as high as you are able), and flex the foot forward. Hold for 2 seconds, then slowly lower. Repeat with your other leg to complete 1 rep.

- **How many:** Repeat 10 times with each leg for 1 set. Rest for 60 seconds, and do a second set. Be careful to avoid pain; reduce or eliminate the ankle weight if necessary.

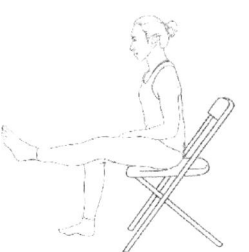

Knee Curls

This will strengthen your hamstrings, which are the big muscles in the back of your thighs, and which help propel you forward and enable you to climb steps and hills.

- **How to:** Again, you'll need ankle weights to provide resistance. Stand with both feet pointed forward, and hold onto a chair back or counter. Slowly curl one leg back and up, as if trying to reach your buttocks with your heel. Hold for 2 seconds, then slowly lower. Repeat with your other leg to complete 1 rep.

- **How many:** Repeat 10 times with each leg for 1 set. Rest for 60 seconds, and do a second set.

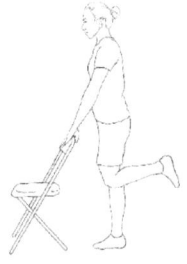

Shifting Weight

Improve your balance while increasing circulation in your legs. Do this anywhere, even while waiting for someone or while on line at the market or bank.

- **How to:** Stand with feet about hip-width apart, and hands at your sides, or lightly touching a chair back or table for balance. Shift your weight to the left and raise your right foot forward a few inches. Hold for 10 seconds, then lower and stand upright.

Repeat by shifting your weight to the right, and lifting your left leg forward and holding for 10 seconds. This is one rep. With practice, extend the hold time up to 30 seconds.

- **How many:** Perform 3 to 6 reps for 1 set. Rest 20 to 30 seconds and do a second set.

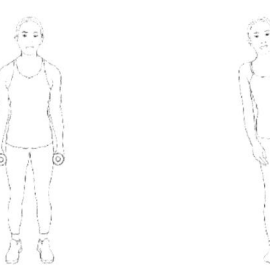

Single Leg Balance

This exercise is identical to the previous shifting weight, but instead of lifting the foot forward, raise the foot to the rear a few inches.

- **How many:** Perform 3 to 6 reps for 1 set. Rest 20 to 30 seconds and do a second set.

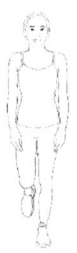

Rock the Boat

This easy movement will improve your balance and coordinate, and strengthen the ankles and feet.

- **How to:** Stand erect with your feet shoulder-width apart. Look straight ahead. Shift your weight onto your right foot and raise your left heel to be standing on the toes of the left foot. Pause. Lower your left heel, and repeat the movement by shifting to the other side, to complete 1 rep.

- **How many:** Alternate shifting side-to-side, and varying the pace as you progress. Do at least 20 reps, rest for 40 seconds, and do a second set.

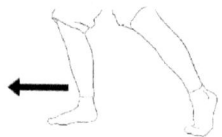

The March

You will engage your quads, hips, glutes, and core, as well as improving balance.

- **How to:** Stand upright with feet about a foot apart. Look ahead. Shift your weight onto your right foot and raise your left knee until your thigh is parallel to the floor. Pause, then lower your foot to the floor.

Shift your weight to the left and repeat the movement by raising your right knee. Raising each leg one time completes 1 rep.

- **How many:** Do at least 10 reps, rest for 40 seconds, and do a second set. As you progress, extend the pause before lowering your legs.

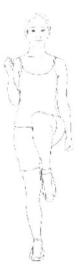 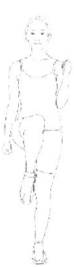

Shoulder Rolls

Loosen and relax your shoulders and extend their range of motion.

- **How to:** Stand erect, with your arms at your sides. Raise your shoulders and roll them forward, down and back, and then back up toward the ears.

- **How many:** Perform 3 or 4 circles in this one direction and then switch, and do the same number of circles in the opposite direction.

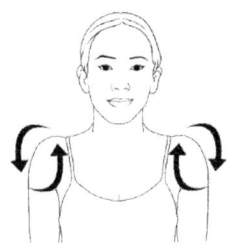

Side Arm Lifts

Loosen and relax your arms and shoulders, and extend their range of motion.

- **How to:** Stand erect, with your arms at your sides. Lift your arms out to the side and raise to shoulder level. Rotate your arms so that your palms face the ceiling. Lower your arms to your sides, and rotate your arms back so your palms face your thighs.

  Try to elevate your arms higher on each lift to the side if you can, according to your shoulders' range of motion.

- **How many:** Continue for the number of repetitions that don't hurt your shoulders.

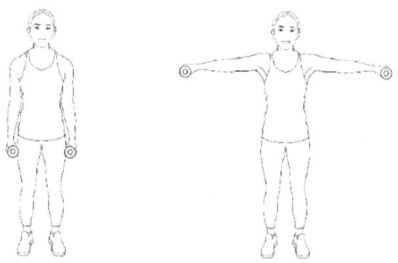

Front Arm Lifts

Loosen and relax your arms and shoulders, and extend their range of motion.

- **How to:** Stand erect, with your arms at your sides. Lift your arms in front of you and raise to shoulder level, with your palms facing each other. Lower your arms to your sides, and rotate your arms back so your palms face your thighs.

Try to elevate your arms higher on each front lift if you can, according to your shoulders' range of motion.

- **How many:** Continue for the number of repetitions that don't hurt your shoulders.

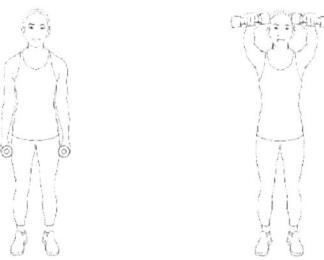

If you read through each of these exercises, you will notice just how easy they are to do. Learn them well, practice them to do them right, and watch your body respond well to your investment of effort.

Weightlifting starter. In the next chapter, you will learn more exercises that you can do with dumbbells.

Chapter 8:

The Dumbbell Exercises

Greater Resistance for Greater Results

You're ready to move up to weights. Now that you know lots of simple bodyweight exercises that you can do at home, it will be an easy transition for you to continue the momentum with the use of dumbbells.

The only equipment you will need are dumbbells because they are quite easy to use and will add some dynamism and greater resistance to your workouts. So, let's get into these dumbbell exercises to add to your 10 week plan.

Hypertrophy

We've referred to hypertrophy previously, but given its importance to building muscle size and strength, this is a good time for a deeper explanation. Hypertrophy is a process of muscle cell growth and increase in size, achieved through certain types of exercise: "When you work out, if you want to tone or improve muscle definition, lifting weights is the most common way to increase hypertrophy" (*Healthline*, 2019).

How it works. Building muscle by lifting weights needs creation of both metabolic fatigue and mechanical damage. When lifting a heavy weight, the "Contractile proteins in the muscles must generate force to overturn the resistance provided by the weight," which results in structural damage to muscle tissues:

- **Metabolic fatigue** occurs when the muscle fibers exhaust the available supply of adenosine triphosphate (ATP), an energy component in the cellular mitochondria that helps muscles to contract. When ATP is depleted, these tiny "energy factories" aren't able to continue to fuel muscular contractions, and are no longer able to lift the weight effectively.

- **Mechanical damage** to muscle cellular proteins triggers a repair response in the body. When damaged fibers in muscle proteins are repaired, the slight overbuilding that occurs results in an increase in the size of the muscle, and its strength.

Both metabolic fatigue and mechanical damage are important for achieving muscular hypertrophy.

There are two kinds of hypertrophy; which to emphasize depends on your fitness objectives:

- **Myofibrillar** hypertrophy is about size; the growth of muscle contraction parts. It will help you to improve strength and speed.

- **Sarcoplasmic** hypertrophy concerns energy; the increased storage of glycogen in muscles. It provides you with greater endurance through sustained energy.

As a general rule, myofibrillar hypertrophy is more effectively achieved by lifting heavier weights for fewer reps, while sarcoplasmic hypertrophy is the result of many reps of lighter weights. You might do 8 to 10 bicep curls with 20 or 25 lbs dumbbells for muscle mass and strength primarily, and endurance secondarily; or 18 to 20 reps using 8 to 10 lbs dumbbells for endurance and speed, and muscle tone and firmness.

How Often to Lift

It's up to you, and depends on your goals and expectations. But whichever option you prefer, remember the importance of rest between weightlifting sessions: Hypertrophy needs time to repair and rebuild your muscle tissues, especially for seniors, whose recovery time is longer. Consider these three options:

- Lifting weights **three** days a week. This allows you one full day between workout sessions to enable your muscles time to recover. But does one day allow sufficient time for a senior to recover? The next option may be preferable and more effective for you.

- Lifting weights **two** days a week. Depending on your age and current fitness level, this may be better for you, especially if you're lifting heavy weights to achieve myofibrillar hypertrophy, and need two or three days of recovery time.

- **Alternating** between upper-body lifting only on one day, and doing only lower-body lifting on a different day. This lets you work different muscles and muscle groups, while allowing sufficient time for rest and recovery. So you can lift weights on 4, 5, 6, and even 7 days a week, as long as specific muscles are not subject to lifting on consecutive days.

Use It or Lose It

That's how the Mayo Clinic (2022) sums up the importance of strength training for seniors, noting that "Lean muscle mass naturally diminishes with age," and further cautioning us that "Your body fat percentage will increase over time if you don't do anything to replace the lean muscle you lose over time." Strength training is what can help you to enhance and to preserve muscle mass and strength at any age.

Here are additional strength training benefits for seniors:

- Strengthen bones. Strength training can reduce the risk of osteoporosis by increasing bone density.

- Manage weight. Strength training can help you to lose some weight, by increasing your metabolism, which burns more calories, both during, and for some time after workouts.

- Enhance quality of life. Strength training can improve your ability to do your usual activities, while protecting your joints and contributing better balance, reducing the risk of falls and helping maintain independence.

- Manage chronic conditions. Strength training can help protect you from heart disease, obesity, arthritis, lower back pain, diabetes and depression.

- Sharpen your thinking skills. In combination, regularly practicing strength training and aerobic exercise can improve learning and thinking skills as you age.

Repetition Maximum

A repetition maximum (RM) is the maximum weight that you are able to lift cleanly, with good form, for a specific number of repetitions. For example, a 10RM would be the heaviest weight you could lift for a set of 10 consecutive reps. Trainers believe that a person's RM is a valid way to measure their strength training progress.

For example, your initial, pre-training RM might be 10 reps of a 10 lb dumbbell. Two weeks later, your RM could progress to 10 reps of a 15 lb weight. Over time, you could keep track as your 10 reps capacity continues to improve.

If your goal is to maximize muscle size and strength, the ideal approach is to keep your RM at 10, and keep upping the weight, and not to increase the reps above 10, and keep lifting the same weight.

One repetition maximum, or 1RM, is also used to measure progress; it's the heaviest weight that you can lift, fully and cleanly, for one time, and only one time. But it has risks of strains, if not done correctly. Follow this procedure for a safe determination of your 1RM:

1. Your muscles that will be challenged must be rested, and not worked hard earlier in the day, or the previous day.

2. Your body needs to be warmed up by doing some light cardio and stretching exercises for 15 to 20 minutes to get your heart and circulation going.

3. The muscles for the 1RM measure need to be warmed up, by doing some reps of a much lighter weight; roughly half of what you expect your 1RM to be. Work, but don't overwork those muscles. Rest for two minutes.

4. Lift a weight that is about 80% of your expected 1RM for three to four reps. Rest for one minute.

5. Increase the weight by 10% and do one rep; rest for one minute, and add another 10% and do 1 rep, if you are able.

6. Keep adding small increments of weight until you can no longer lift the weight fully. The previous weight that you were able to lift for one full rep is your 1RM.

The Dumbbell Exercises

These are the classics that have been used to build muscle and strength for generations. Resist lifting and lowering the dumbbells too fast, as the momentum weakens the resistance. Exhale as you lift, and inhale as you lower.

Be careful. Select weights that you can lift around 10 reps (8 to 12) for each of 3 sets; the last 1 or 2 reps should be tough, but just doable. Start carefully; don't lift weights that are too heavy when starting out.

The Chest Exercise

This exercise will engage the deltoid muscle in your shoulders, giving you greater ability to lift and carry.

- **How to:** Stand erect, with a straight back, holding a dumbbell in each hand at your sides, with knuckles pointing forward. Raise the dumbbells to your head, pause for one second, then lower the dumbbells back down to your hips

Exhale as you raise the weights, and inhale as you lower. You can also raise each arm alternately.

- **How many:** Do 3 sets of 8 to 12 reps, with 45 to 60 seconds rest between sets.

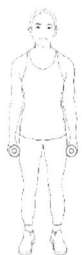 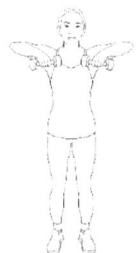

Bent-Over Rows

This targets muscles in your mid and upper back, and works the chest's pectorals and upper arm's brachialis, and activates the shoulder rotator cuff muscles.

- **How to:** Stand with your legs shoulder-width apart, and with your knees slightly bent. Hold a dumbbell in each hand with the palms facing your body. Bend to a 45-degree angle, keeping your back straight.

    Exhale as you lift the weights straight up to parallel with your shoulders; or slightly lower. Lower without pausing to the starting position.

- **How many:** Do 3 sets of 8 to 12 reps, with 45 to 60 seconds rest between sets.

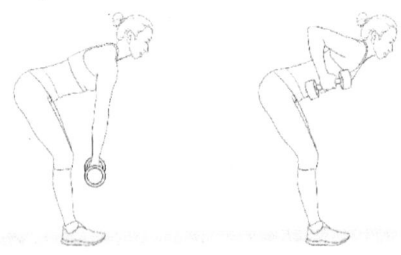

Dumbbell Front Raise

Building shoulder muscle strength is the primary function of this dumbbell lift, which works the rotator cuff group.

- **How to:** Stand erect, with your back straight, holding a dumbbell in each hand at your sides, with knuckles pointing forward. Keep your arms straight (slight elbow bend is okay) as you raise the dumbbells, arcing upwards and outwards until close to parallel to the floor.

  Then lower the dumbbells back down to your sides. Exhale as you raise the weights, and inhale as you lower. You can also raise each arm alternately.

- **How many:** Do 3 sets of 8 to 12 reps, with 45 to 60 seconds rest between sets.

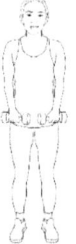
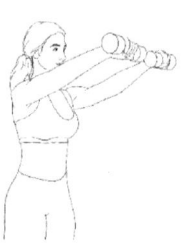

Bicep Curls

This is the classic exercise to strengthen the upper arms, especially the biceps, and secondarily, the brachialis and brachioradialis muscles in your lower arms.

- **How to:** Stand upright, with your arms fully extended at your sides, and holding a dumbbell in each hand. Your palms should face forward. Slowly raise the weight toward your shoulders, reaching as far as you can, then lowering the weight back to your sides. Exhale as you raise the dumbbells; inhale as you lower.

- **How many:** Do 3 sets of 8 to 12 reps, with 45 to 60 seconds rest between sets.

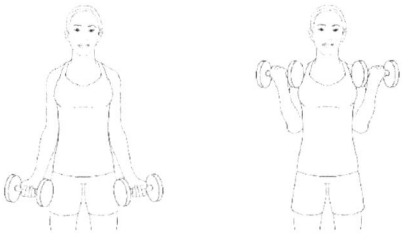

Dumbbell Triceps

The triceps brachii are the muscles in the back of your upper arms; they connect from the elbow to the latissimus dorsi, and come into play when lifting and pushing.

- **How to:** Stand or sit upright with a dumbbell in each hand. Raise the dumbbells to the sides of your head, pause, then raise them up toward the ceiling, and bend your elbows to lower the weights toward the backs of your shoulders. You should feel the tension in your triceps. Pause, then raise the weights upward, and then back to the sides of your head. This completes 1 rep.

- **How many:** Do 3 sets of 10 reps, with 30 to 40 seconds rest between sets.

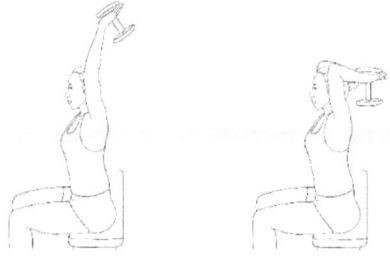

Dumbbell Leg Lunge

This is a version of lunges, but with weights to increase the resistance. The quads which connect the hips to the knees, and steady the kneecap, are the primary beneficiaries, along with hips and glutes. The quads help you stand, climb, and cycle.

- **How to:** Stand holding dumbbells in each hand, arms relaxed, at your sides. Take a long stride forward so your thighs are parallel to the floor. Don't let the knee of the forward leg extend past the toes of the rear foot. Pause, then return to the starting upright position. Repeat the movement with your other leg.

- **How many:** Do 1 set of 10 lunges with each leg; rest for 60 seconds, then do 1 more set. If your knees hurt during the lunge, don't extend downward as far.

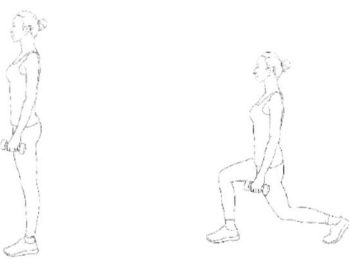

Dumbbell Squat

Similar to the dumbbell lunges, this is a version of squats, with weights to increase the resistance. This too strengthens your quads, along with hips and glutes.

- **How to:** Stand holding dumbbells in each hand, arms relaxed, at your sides. Bend forward slightly at the hips, but keep your back straight and squat down until your thighs are parallel to the floor. Pause, then rise back up to the starting upright position.

- **How many:** Do 1 set of 10 squats; rest for 60 seconds, then do 1 or 2 more sets. If your knees hurt during the squat, don't extend downward as deeply.

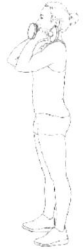 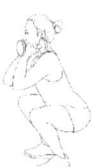

Dumbbell Chest Press

The chest press uses the resistance from the weights to strengthen your pecs and other chest muscles, along with your lats at the upper sides and back, and your shoulders.

- **How to:** Hold a dumbbell in each hand, and lie on an exercise bench, if you have one, or on the floor (use a yoga mat or carpet for cushioning), or even with your upper back on a large exercise ball. Hold the weights with knuckles facing forward, close to your chest; just in front of your shoulders.

Begin by exhaling and raising the dumbbells straight up to the ceiling until your arms are fully extended. Pause, then inhale and lower to the starting position.

- **How many:** Do 1 set of 10 to 12 presses, rest for 60 seconds, then do 1 or 2 more sets.

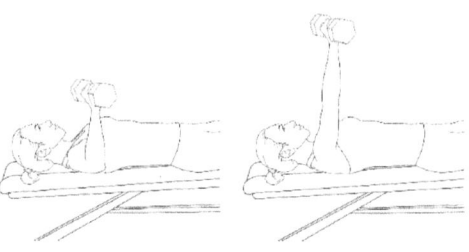

Dumbbell Pullover

You'll strengthen your upper back, shoulders, pecs, and triceps with this classic dumbbell lift.

- **How to:** This exercise can be performed on a bench, the floor (cushioned with a mat or carpet), or an exercise ball. Lie on your back with just one dumbbell on the floor near your head (where you can reach it). Grasp the dumbbell with both hands, and raise it toward the ceiling.

    Begin by lowering the weight in an arc to the floor behind your head. Pause momentarily, then follow the same arc to the upward starting position.

- **How many:** Do 1 set of 10 to 12 lowering and raising cycles, rest for 60 seconds, then do 1 or 2 more sets.

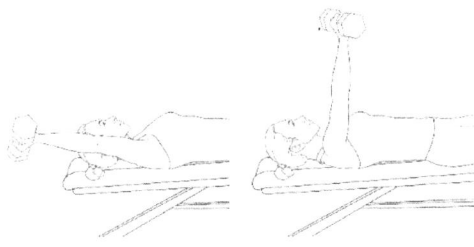

Standing Calf Raise

This weighted version of regular calf raises increases the resistance to build your calf muscles, and strengthen your feet and ankle joints. This will improve your stride.

- **How to:** Stand erect with a dumbbell in each hand, arms at your sides. Rise up on your toes as high as you can and pause for one second, then slowly lower your heels to the floor. You can vary the intensity by increasing the weight, or by extending how long you pause at the top of each calf raise. If balance is a concern, you can shift the weights a little.

- **How many:** You may do up to 20 reps in each of 3 sets, if the weights you're holding allow; otherwise do as many as you comfortably are able.

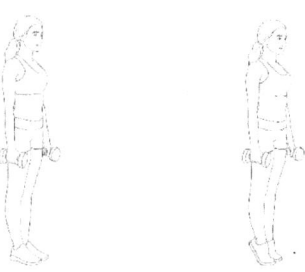

Deadlift

A deadlift is any movement that involves bending over to lift something. When dumbbells are involved, and good form and posture is maintained, there are strengthening benefits to your hamstrings, glutes, lats, core, and lower back.

- **How to:** Stand, holding the dumbbells in front of your thighs, and with your palms facing your body, and with your knees relaxed. Begin slowly lowering the weights by tightening your core, bending your knees, and pushing your butt back. Be careful to keep your back straight as you lower the dumbbells to your shins. Pause, then slowly raise back up to the starting position.

- **How many:** Perform 1 set of 10 to 12 reps, rest, then do 1 or 2 more sets.

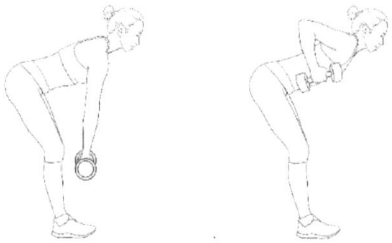

Scaption

This is one of the easier ways to strengthen your shoulders and increase their range of motion. Just be sure the weights are not too heavy; start light to avoid discomfort or strain.

- **How to:** Stand holding dumbbells in each hand, arms relaxed, at your sides, and palms turned in, toward your body. Raise the weights at a 45 degree angle (midway between front and side) and with arms fully extended. Elevate the weights to just above shoulder height, then lower to the starting position. Don't lift and lower too fast; slower movement is more beneficial.

- **How many:** Do 1 set of 12 to 16 reps; rest and do 1 or 2 more sets.

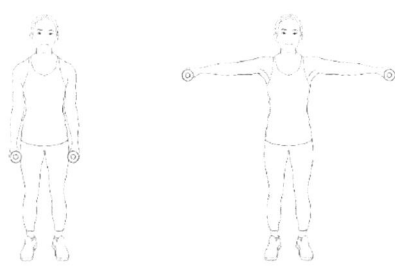

Dumbbell Row

To improve your posture, and relieve lower back pain, dumbbell rows are used to tighten your core and the muscles that support your spine and shoulder blades.

- **How to:** Stand with feet apart, holding the dumbbells at your sides, with palms turned toward your body. Tighten your core, push your butt back and hinge forward at the hips so your body is at a 45 degree angle.

  Keep your back straight and lower the weight with your arms fully extended. Begin by squeezing your shoulder blades together, bending your elbows and pull the weights up to your lower abdomen; pause, then lower the weights back down to the starting position.

- **How many:** Perform 8 to 10 reps or until exhaustion; rest 60 seconds, do a second set, rest, and a third set.

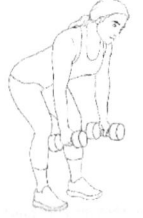 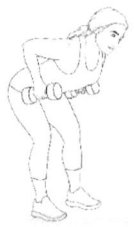

Seated Shoulder Overhead Press

The shoulders tend to weaken as we age, and are subject to strains and tears, especially the rotator cuff muscles. This press will restore lost strength, and also build the triceps.

- **How to:** Sit in a chair and slide your hips and back against the backrest. Hold a dumbbell in each hand, and raise it to shoulder height; your elbows should be extended to the sides, and your hands positioned so your palms face forward. Raise the weights upward toward the ceiling, until your arms are fully extended, but don't lock your elbows. Then lower the weights to the shoulder-level starting position to complete 1 rep.

- **How many:** Do a first set of 10 to 12 reps, and rest for 40 to 60 seconds, and do a second set. If your shoulders feel okay and there's no pain, rest for 60 seconds and perform a third set.

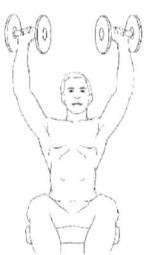

Now you have the fully-fledged guide on all the exercises you can do at home, using your own bodyweight as explained in the previous chapter, or a set of dumbbells, for all the resistance you need to build muscles, and become appreciably stronger.

Tips and tricks. This is a good time to finetune your understanding of building and strengthening your muscles; the advice that follows will help you to exercise the right way, the safe way, and the most productive way.

Chapter 9:

Lifting Methods and Tips

More Ways to Build Muscle and Grow Stronger

You are not limited in the range of exercises you can do, in addition to those you have already learned. There are alternatives and variations that will create the resistance you need to achieve positive results.

Lifting can be challenging, and even risky, if you aren't aware of what you need to do, and the correct way to do it. This applies whether the lifting is done with bodyweight or dumbbells to provide resistance.

Since all the exercises you have learned in the previous chapters explain "how to" and "how many" in detail, what you need now are some tips on lifting techniques that can help you perfect your performance.

Additional Lifting Methods

There are many ways to provide the resistance you need to initiate hypertrophy and make you stronger, with bigger, firmer muscles. Your muscles don't care if you are working out in a gym or fitness center, or at home. Here are examples of additional methods you can consider as your preferred way to get stronger.

Method #1: Resistance Bands

We've referred briefly to these stretchable elastic bands as a very low cost option as far as resistance "equipment" is concerned, and noted they can be carried easily to use at work or when traveling.

Do not underestimate the potential muscle and strength-building power these simple, lightweight bands offer. Resistance is resistance, regardless of the source; what matters is how it is used. Fortunately, you just need to emulate the weightlifting and bodyweight movements they are replacing.

Note: How many reps you perform depends on the resistance of the bands you are using, and since this can vary, do sufficient reps in each of 3 sets so that the last few reps are tough to do, while maintaining good form.

Bicep Curl

Your upper arms, especially the biceps at the front, will be the primary beneficiaries of this simulation of the classic curl. Shoulders, upper back, and forearms also benefit.

- **How to:** Instead of lifting a dumbbell from hip to shoulder, stand with your right foot on a looped band, and hold the opposite end in your right hand, with your arm fully extended downward, and your palm facing upward. Choose a band that has tension when held at hip level; if necessary, adjust the length by shifting your foot to tighten the band.

Curl your right hand slowly up toward your shoulder, keeping your upper arm and elbow close to your body. Pause for a moment, then slowly lower your hand to the starting position, to complete one rep. You may also exercise both arms by placing both feet on the bottom of the loop, and grasping the loop at the top, with hands placed palms up, and shoulder width apart.

- **How many:** Do sufficient reps in each of 3 sets so that the last few reps are tough to do. As with dumbbell curls, keep good upright posture.

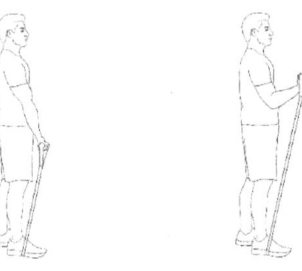

Triceps Press

You should feel good tension in your triceps, shoulders and lats.

- **How to:** Place the resistance band loop on a doorknob and grasp the other end of the loop with both hands. Raise your hands with palms facing upward to the level of your head; adjust the length of the band so there is some tension at this point (for example, shorten it by wrapping a few extra loops around the doorknob).

Begin the movement by pressing upward to fully extend your arms, but don't lock your elbows; pause, then slowly lower your hands to head level, to do one rep.

- **How many:** Do 2 or 3 sets of as many reps as you need.

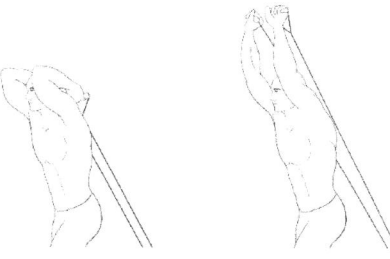

Overhead Pulldown

Your chest, lats, and upper back will benefit from this simulation of pull up, or a pulldown machine at a gym.

- **How to:** Reach up to place the resistance band loop over the top of a door, so it rests a few inches forward of the door edge. With both hands, grasp the loop high enough to have some tension when you begin to pull downward.

  Turn your hands so the palms are facing downward, and begin the movement by pulling down toward your chest, or below if possible. Pause, and slowly let your hands rise to the starting position; this is 1 rep.

- **How many:** Do 2 or 3 sets of as many reps as you need. Tip: You can increase the tension by squatting down slightly to increase the stretch.

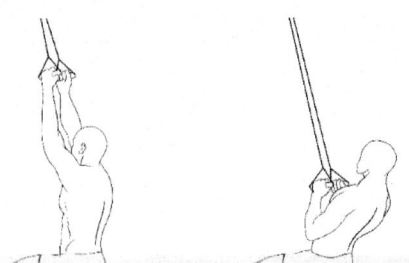

Wall Push Up

Your arms, shoulders, chest, upper back and core benefit from this intensified push up against a wall.

- **How to:** You can increase the resistance of wall push ups by placing a band behind your shoulders and upper back, and pressing the ends of the band against the wall when you are in the "down" or forward position, with your head close to the wall.

  Ensure that the band is able to provide resistance as you push up to begin the movement, and be careful not to place the band behind your neck.

- **How many:** Do 2 or 3 sets of as many reps as you need to make the last few reps hard to do.

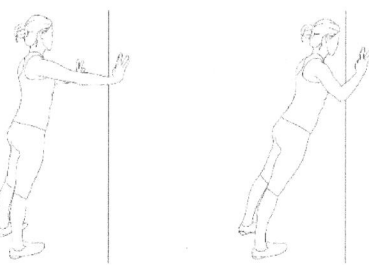

Method #2: Isometrics

Unlike almost all other forms of exercise and strength building, isometrics involve creating tension without movement. The tension is created by a full contraction of the muscles that occurs when they are fully challenged; with isometrics, the contraction is extended. According to *Insider* (2020), "An isometric is when you hold the portion of a lift for anywhere from a few seconds to a minute (or more)."

For example, during a dumbbell row, "Hold the extended arms part of the lift for 10 seconds to feel a stretch in your lats." This increases the time that your muscles are working at close to maximum effort.

Here are two examples of isometric exercises that you can perform without weights; let these inspire you to think of other bodyweight exercises you can do with the *extended pauses* at the moment of *maximum resistance*:

- **Upper body.** Try this: While standing or sitting, place the palms of your hands together a few inches in front of your chest. Now press the palms together as hard as you can, extend your elbows out to the sides, and hold the tension for 5 or 6 seconds, then release. Wait 20 to 30 seconds, then repeat the pressing, rest again, and repeat a third time.

    This isometric strengthens and tones your pec, shoulders, triceps, forearms, and wrists. For it to be effective, be sure your pressure is intense.

    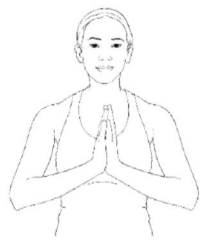

- **Lower body.** Try this: Stand with your feet about shoulder width apart, hold your arms slightly upward and forward for balance, and squat down until your thighs are horizontal to the floor.

    But instead of rising right back up, hold the squat for 6 or 8 seconds (or longer, if you can), and then rise to the upright starting position. Rest for 20 seconds, then repeat the cycle 2 or 3 more times. If your knees hurt, don't squat as deeply.

These isometric squats will build your thighs, especially the quads upfront, and will strengthen the muscles that control your knee joints.

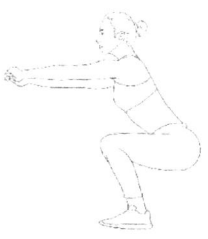

Method #3: Deadlifts

- **Towel leg curls.** This is a no-equipment alternative to hamstring curls; it's like a push up for the upper legs. Lie on your back on a smooth floor (not a mat or carpet this time), and place a towel or similar heavy fabric about two feet ahead of your hips. Now raise your knees and place your feet on the towel. Begin the exercise by pressing down on the fabric while you pull your feet back to your butt.

  Without pausing, keep the downward pressure as you push the towel forward to the starting position, to complete 1 rep. Do about 10 to 12 reps; pause for a minute, and do 1 or 2 more sets.

It's the combination of downward pressure and pulling and pushing that creates the resistance. Your hamstrings and glutes are the primary beneficiaries.

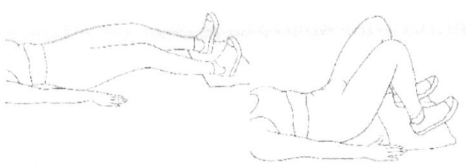

Banded pull-through. Here's another way to work and strengthen your hamstrings and glutes without using weights or a machine; just a resistance band. Attach a long looped band to the bottom of a pole, or the leg of a dresser or heavy table. Stand with your back to the pole or table, and as you hold onto the band, step over it with one leg so you can grasp the band with both hands, and hold it between your legs

- Hinge forward at the hips and flex your knees so your body is bent at a 45 degree angle (at least); be sufficiently forward for there to be some tension in the band. Begin the exercise by raising your body to the upright position, while keeping your hands and the band between your legs. Pause, then bend back down to the starting position.

- Depending on the resistance of the band, do between 12 and 20 reps, rest for 40 seconds, and repeat 1 more set. (If 20 reps does not make you tired, step forward to increase the resistance).

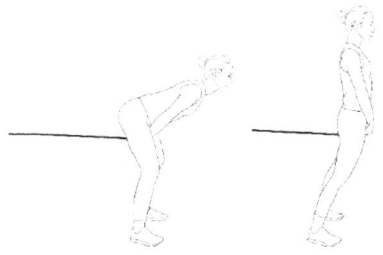

Method #4: Barbells

Barbell press. Think about a barbell press, also called a chest press, in which you lie on your back on a bench, and press (push) a barbell up toward the ceiling to fully extend your arms. Now think about a push up, and you'll realize it's the same, only in reverse.

A push up lifts about 65% of your body weight, so if you weigh 160 lbs, your push up is like pressing 104 lbs. You can calculate using your own weight, but even at a weight of 100 lbs, that's the same as pressing 65 lbs. And doing push ups doesn't pose the risks of dropping the barbell! Do 3 sets of 12 reps, or the number of reps that you can just do.

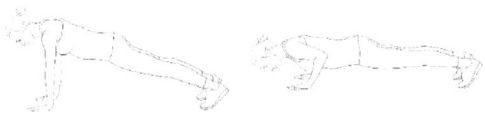

Barbell rows. Can you replicate the barbell row workout of bending forward and pulling a barbell up to your body? A simple set of movements called "**Y-T-W**" can get the job done. "This simple exercise uses all the same shoulder and upper back muscles that a barbell row would activate," *Insider* reports.

Lie on your stomach on a mat or carpet, with legs extended, and your arms fully extended about 8 inches from the sides of your head, so you are in a "Y" shape, seen from above. Begin by raising your arms up and down for 10 pulses. Then create the "T" shape by extending your arms to the sides, and repeat the 10 lifting pulses. Finally, slide your arms toward your hips to form a "W" and perform 10 more pulses. Relax, then repeat 1 or 2 more times.

Barbell overheads. Unlike the previous two exercises, this one requires a weight you can lift with one hand to give the same results, or a bit more, as barbell overhead presses. Stand erect, with your feet apart, holding a dumbbell or kettle weight in one hand at your side. Hoist the weight up to head level, then extend your arm up toward the ceiling. Reach as high as you can without locking your elbow. Pause for 1 second, then lower the weight to head level to complete 1 rep.

In addition to strengthening your shoulders, chest, upper arms, and lats, by standing you will also create tension in your core, and obliques on the opposite side. Do 1 set of 10 reps, and repeat with the other arm. Do 2 more sets with each arm, resting for 30 seconds between sets.

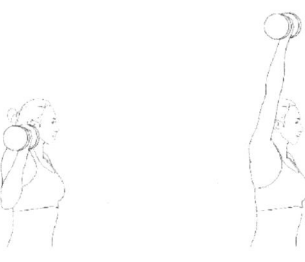

Strength Training Tips

Throughout the exercise instructions there have been tips for effectiveness and to avoid injuries; this section will recap some of the most important points.

1. **How often.** Strength train at least 2 times every week. It's important to rest each muscle group before the next workout, but don't rest two long. Ideally, as a senior you should allow 2 days of rest before returning the same muscles, but no more than 3 or 4 days if your strengthening and muscle-building is to progress.

2. **Joint care.** Be kind to your joints and keep them safe. You can risk abrading the calcium that lines the joints for lubricity, resulting in grinding, and pain, as with runner's knee or elbow injuries. Be careful lifting and stretching too, since the tendons and ligaments that connect muscles to joints cannot bounce back with resilience, like muscles can.

3. **Start carefully.** It's a good idea to start your strengthening program with exercises that use bodyweight for resistance, instead of free weights like dumbbells; you're much less likely to overlift and end up straining a muscle or a joint. Even if you've moved on to weights, work the targeted muscle groups with stretching and light bodyweight lift and pushing, like

squats, lunges, wall push ups, dips, and shoulder stretches holding a very light weight, even a water bottle.

4. **Rest and recover.** Plan for extra recovery time; as noted in the first tip. Your muscles need 2 or even 3 days of recovery for hypertrophy to repair and rebuild the muscle fibers and cells that are damaged during the workouts. You can do strength training every day, as long as the same muscle groups are not being worked on consecutive days, or with only 1 day of rest.

5. **Warm up.** Your muscles and your heart will thank you if you take a little time to warm up and get your circulation going before doing serious resistance training. About 10 to 15 minutes of light cardio, on the treadmill or outdoors, for example, plus some light stretching should help increase the blood delivery of oxygen and nutrients to all the muscles. Some reps of lighter weights are also helpful to warm up before the heavy weights are used.

6. **Alert to pain.** Any intense workout, including weightlifting, can feel difficult, but you should not feel pain; if you do, stop what you are doing. You may experience soreness, especially the next day, but a sharp pain, especially in a joint, is your body's signal that something's wrong. Chest pain, especially during a cardio workout, can mean your heart is not receiving enough oxygen, and you need to stop and get it checked out with your doctor.

7. **Breathe.** Don't hold your breath during exercise; you want your body to function normally, and keep supplying the oxygen that the muscles urgently need when being contracted to lift weights. The correct way to breathe during strength training is to inhale during

the release, or weight lowering half of each rep, and to exhale during the lifting, strenuous half of the rep.

8. **Posture.** Always be aware of your form and posture when you exercise, so that the movement is performed correctly, and you avoid straining your back or other areas. A common mistake is to hunch forward when doing biceps curls with weights or bands, which shortens the arc of the lift, and puts strain on the upper, thoracic spine. A straight spine during lifts will be an injury-free spine.

9. **Don't lock.** Keeping the joints of your arms and legs from locking during extension avoids risking strains and sprains. Pause at the top of arm extensions just before the elbows lock, and when you stand upright after bending or squatting, be careful not to lock your knees.

10. **Better balance.** As we mature, our sense of balance diminishes, making us a bit clumsier, but also more likely to fall, which can lead to serious injuries. We also lose flexibility, as tendons and ligaments stiffen. Improve your balance by standing on one foot, and slightly raising the other. Also try raising one knee to hip height, hold for 15 seconds, then reversing legs. Once you get good at this, try with eyes closed.

Planning. Stay safe and learn to lift the proper ways. You can use other methods of lifting including bodyweight calisthenics and resistance bands instead of dumbbells or barbells.

You may do these exercises at your own pace, as long as you remember to take your time and pace yourself, and keep up the momentum by following a schedule, like the worksheet for a 10 week plan that you can do to bring strength back to your life; it's coming up in the next chapter.

Chapter 10:

The 10-Week Plan

Planning Will Make the Difference for You

This 10-week plan can really make starting easier for you, and will keep your progress on track. The simple worksheets let you tick off when you are done each day, and are designed to keep you motivated and keep your workouts organized. Another benefit is inclusiveness: You won't have to depend on your memory to ensure you are including all of the exercises you want in your strength training program.

Discipline yourself to commit to the scheduled workouts, so take your time organizing your plan, study them, and don't overextend yourself. Have fun knowing you're on your way to building muscle mass and getting stronger!

Be flexible! These schedules can be changed as your preference changes, and don't worry if you miss a day—consider it an additional recovery day. Just be sure to adjust the schedule so you don't end up pushing two similar workout days together.

The schedules which follow are presented as example, but feel free to create your own plans, based on your needs:

- One person might want a total body workout during each session, which will limit resistance training to 2 or 3 days a week.

- Another could prefer to do strength training almost every day by concentrating on just the upper body on one day, core and midbody on the next day, and hips, glutes, and legs on the third day.

- To repeat the point: Just be sure not to do resistance training with the same muscles on consecutive days.; give hypertrophy the time it needs to rebuild.

- The following section will reinforce the amounts of sets and reps you should be doing during each workout.

Reps and Sets

While you've seen many references to reps and sets so far in the instructions, it's worth taking a few moments to confirm the definitions and applications to your workouts:

- **Reps** are repetitions; the number of times you perform a complete cycle of an exercise. When you curl a pair of dumbbells from your hips to your shoulders, and then lower the weight back down to the starting point (your hips), that is one rep. The same goes for every lifting exercise, with or without weights: One down-and-up of a push up is 1 rep.

- **Sets** are a continuous series of reps that are performed without stopping. If you curl (raise and lower) the dumbbells for 10 consecutive reps, that is 1 set. When you then rest for 30 or 60 seconds, and repeat the cycle of curls, that makes it 2 sets. Do it one more time after the rest and it's a 3rd set.

- **How many** reps and sets depends on you and the amount of weight you are lifting. There are many options, but the go-to standard for most trainers is for you to do 8 to 10 reps of a weight that you can just lift about 10 times before having to stop, and assuming your posture and form remain good, and you're not jerking the weight to get it up fully.

  A total of 3 sets is typically recommended, but let your body tell you if you're up to it.

  For bodyweight and resistance band exercises, it's hard to select a specific weight, so let exhaustion be your guide by doing enough reps to tire yourself without straining. The same total of 3 sets applies here as well.

- **Be cautious.** Safety reminders keep coming up on these pages, because injuries can occur when weights that are too heavy are lifted, or dropped, or if warning pains are ignored. When in doubt, use a lighter weight and do a few more reps, instead of lifting a weight you may lose control of, or cause a strain.

  Do not be tempted to keep up with others in a gym, who are stronger; give yourself time to build your strength.

Weekly Schedules

The following schedules are suggestive, and are designed to take you through most of the many basic and dumbbell exercises, so you can experience them before focusing on those you prefer to do regularly. They begin with just 4 exercises in a day, and have you up to 8 later on, as you grow stronger and build endurance.

Check the boxes as appropriate to keep track of what you've done.

Week 1   *Date:*

Exercise	Day 1	Day 2	Day 3	Day 4	Day 5	Day 6	Day 7
Rest Day*							
	8 to 12 Reps — 3 Sets						
Squats to Chair							
Wall Push Ups							
DB** Front Raise							
DB** Leg Lunge							

*Rest Day = No resistance exercise but good for cardio like brisk walking, jogging, cycling, swimming, active gardening and other activities that raise your pulse.

**DB = Dumbbell exercise. You may substitute similar basic bodyweight or stretch band exercises if you don't have access to weights.

Week 2   *Date:*

Exercise	Day 1	Day 2	Day 3	Day 4	Day 5	Day 6	Day 7
Rest Day							
	8 to 12 Reps — 3 Sets							
Wall Angels							
Pec Stretches							
DB Chest Exercise							
DB Bent Over Rows							

Exercise	Day 1	Day 2	Day 3	Day 4	Day 5	Day 6	Day 7

Week 3   *Date:*

Exercise	Day 1	Day 2	Day 3	Day 4	Day 5	Day 6	Day 7
Rest Day							
	8 to 12 Reps — 3 Sets							
Pelvic Tilts							
Shoulder Blade Squeeze							

Exercise	Day 1	Day 2	Day 3	Day 4	Day 5	Day 6	Day 7
Heel Raises							
DB Curls							
DB Pullover							

Week 4 *Date:*

Exercise	Day 1	Day 2	Day 3	Day 4	Day 5	Day 6	Day 7
Rest Day							
	8 to 12 Reps — 3 Sets						
Toe Taps							

Exercise	Day 1	Day 2	Day 3	Day 4	Day 5	Day 6	Day 7
Finger Marching							
Wall Push Ups							
DB Calf Raise							
DB Deadlift							

Week 5   *Date:*

Exercise	Day 1	Day 2	Day 3	Day 4	Day 5	Day 6	Day 7
Rest Day							

Exercise	Day 1	Day 2	Day 3	Day 4	Day 5	Day 6	Day 7
	8 to 12 Reps — 3 Sets							
Knee Lifts							
Shoulder Rolls							
Wall Angels							
DB Scaption							
DB Row							

Week 6   Date:

Exercises	Day 1	Day 2	Day 3	Day 4	Day 5	Day 6	Day 7

Exercises	Day 1	Day 2	Day 3	Day 4	Day 5	Day 6	Day 7
Rest Day							
	8 to 12 Reps — 3 Sets						
Rock the Boat							
Side Arm Lifts							
Pec Stretches							
DB Seated Shoulder Press							
DB Leg Lunge							

Week 7   *Date:*

Exercises	Day 1	Day 2	Day 3	Day 4	Day 5	Day 6	Day 7
Rest Day							
	8 to 12 Reps — 3 Sets							
Knee Curls							
Front Arm Lifts							
Side Hip Raise							
Toe Taps							
DB Triceps							
DB Leg Lunge							
DB Scaption							

Week 8   Date:

Exercises	Day 1	Day 2	Day 3	Day 4	Day 5	Day 6	Day 7
Rest Day							
	8 to 12 Reps — 3 Sets						
Step Ups							
Wall Slides							
Pelvic Tilts							
Finger Marching							
DB Chest							
DB Bent Over Rows							
DB Front Raise							

Week 9 *Date:*

Exercises	Day 1	Day 2	Day 3	Day 4	Day 5	Day 6	Day 7
Rest Day							
	8 to 12 Reps — 3 Sets						
Chest Exercise							
Toe Stands							
Shoulder Blade Squeeze							
Heel Raises							
DB Bicep Curls							
DB Leg Lunge							
DB Squat							
DB Deadlift							

Exercises	Day 1	Day 2	Day 3	Day 4	Day 5	Day 6	Day 7

Week 10   *Date:*

Exercises	Day 1	Day 2	Day 3	Day 4	Day 5	Day 6	Day 7
Rest Day							
	8 to 12 Reps — 3 Sets						
Standing Balance							
Quadruped Opposite Arm							
Finger Marching							
Chin Up							
DB Triceps							
DB Chest Press							

Exercises	Day 1	Day 2	Day 3	Day 4	Day 5	Day 6	Day 7
DB Pullover							
DB Calf Raise							

Total Body Schedule

This 10 day total body schedule allows you to perform resistance training on some consecutive days while ensuring 2 rest days for the upper and lower body muscle groups. You may do cardio on all days if you prefer; especially on days when no resistance training is done, as in days 3, 6, and 9 in this example:

10 Day - Total Body   *Date:*

Exercise	Day 1	Day 2	Day 3	Day 4	Day 5	Day 6	Day 7	Day 8	Day 9	Day 10
Upper Body 8 to 12 Reps — 3 Sets											
	☐		☐		☐		☐			

Exercise	Day 1	Day 2	Day 3	Day 4	Day 5	Day 6	Day 7	Day 8	Day 9	Day 10
Pec Stretches										
DB Chest Exercise		Rest	Rest		Rest	Rest		Rest	Rest	
DB Bicep Curls										

Lower Body 8 to 12 Reps — 3 Sets

Step Ups										
Toe Stands					Rest		Rest			Rest
DB Leg										

Exercise	Day 1	Day 2	Day 3	Day 4	Day 5	Day 6	Day 7	Day 8	Day 9	Day 10
Lunge		☐	☐		☐			☐		
DB Squat		☐	☐		☐			☐		

Check the boxes as appropriate to keep track of what you've done.

Chapter 11:

Strength Training FAQs

Gain Confidence With Knowledge

With all this information on physical conditioning coming your way, you might be feeling a tad overwhelmed, and maybe a bit hesitant to continue with this journey. If that sounds like you, this final chapter will answer some of the most frequently asked questions you may have about strength training, and give you more confidence to begin your training with enthusiasm.

I haven't exercised in years, why should I start?

- It's never too late to benefit. According to the American Council on Exercise (ACE), "Even if you've never been active, it's never too late to reap the many health benefits of regular exercise." Regular cardiovascular exercise, including brisk walking, jogging, ellipticals, cycling, and swimming can strengthen the heart and circulatory system.

- "Strength exercise, or resistance training, helps preserve muscle tissue and bone health" (ACE, 2005). In combination, cardio and resistance exercise increases energy and endurance. "It also helps control blood sugar and cholesterol levels and works as a natural mood elevator."

Can I exercise if I have a medical condition?

- Play it safe. It's best practice, and responsible, to get checked out with your healthcare provider before starting any exercise program. Your doctor will want to check your heart and any health problems you may have, and may recommend certain exercises for your specific condition, as well as more beneficial for you.

- "Regular exercise helps manage health conditions and can speed up the recovery process of serious illnesses, including heart attack, stroke and joint-replacement surgery," ACE advises.

How much exercise is enough?

- The amount of exercise you will do depends on your objectives, and the condition your body is in. If you are a senior who is just starting strength training, it's best that you start with moderation; the 10-week plan in the previous chapter is designed to take things slowly so that you can test the waters, while progressing, week after week.

- As we've explained, do not lift weights that are too heavy; work your way up in weight gradually to reach your strength goals. Remember the importance of rest, and never work the same muscle groups on consecutive days.

If I don't have a weight problem, do I need to exercise?

- Strength training is much more than losing weight. "Even if your weight is in a healthy range, regular exercise is key for maintaining good health and to reduce health risks," ACE notes, citing a study that discovered "Physically fit overweight people had significantly lower health risks than thin, sedentary people."

- Resistance exercise strengthens you physically while improving your mobility, balance, and enhancing your lifestyle. Keeping in good shape will also help keep your weight down, and avoid the annual weight gains that happen after we turn 50, and our metabolisms slow down and burn fewer calories

Will strength training cost a lot of money?

- It's actually quite the opposite: The strength training programs that you've learned in this book can easily be done at home with or without equipment. For example, bodyweight strength training can be performed with only a mat or carpet to lie on, and furniture or a counter to lean on.

- If you prefer to lift weights, a set of dumbbells with adjustable weights is all you need, and also you have the popular option of very low cost stretchable resistance bands to replicate the weightlifting exercises.

- The Mediterranean diet presented to you is simple, and can be followed using very affordable, yet healthy ingredients.

Is strength training too hard for someone of my age?

- You are never too old to build muscles and strength; in fact, it becomes more important as you age, to compensate for the gradual reduction in muscle mass that occurs naturally in all of us: "Adults lose 4-6 lbs. of muscle tissue per decade, which means a significant loss of body strength and a lower resting metabolism," ACE reports.

- As long as you start slowly and use minimal weights to work up gradually, you will safely reverse the loss of muscle, and the loss of strength and overall ability that comes with it.

- The importance of rest for repair and rebuilding of muscle tissues goes doubly for seniors: Don't work the same muscle group on consecutive days. If you find that your max weight is too strenuous, cut it back a few pounds, and increase the reps. There is no age restriction, so start exercising today.

How often should I train?

- If you want a total body workout during each session, plan on skipping at least a day in-between each session; 2 to 3 sessions per week, ideally. You can do strength training more often, even daily, if you rotate muscle groups. For example, the upper body on Monday; the lower body on Tuesday; cardio-only on Wednesday, then repeat.

- Use the 10-week plan in the previous chapter for guidance, knowing you can customize which muscle groups to work, and choose the specific exercises to perform. Don't rush yourself; patience will get you strong and keep you safe.

What is the best exercise for me?

- This is up to you, and depends on what parts of your body you are targeting and what types of exercise you are most comfortable with. As for the type of exercise, bodyweight calisthenics require no equipment, can be done anywhere and any time, and are less likely to cause injury. Weightlifting requires that you have access to a set of variable weight dumbbells, but may produce results a bit faster.

- Elastic stretch bands come close to replicating weightlifting, and can also intensify bodyweight movements. Which specific exercises you choose—you have instructions for 26 bodyweight and 14 dumbbell movements to consider—so it's a matter of matching your goals with the most appropriate exercises.

Is strength training really safe for me to do?

- Absolutely! It's highly beneficial and risk-free if you follow the safety tips that have been explained, and are attentive to what you are doing as you do it: Be mindful and you'll be aware of your form and posture, as well as noting any strains or pains that might signal a problem.

- To repeat, if you have been sedentary and are out of condition, see your doctor for clearance and recommended types of exercise before getting into lifting. You are unique, and what's good for others may not be appropriate for you.

You've made it! Your strengthening education is complete. On to the Conclusion.

Conclusion

This is Your Time: Use It Well

How are you feeling now? You should be proud to have taken the important step in your commitment to getting into great physical condition by reading *Strength Training for Seniors*. But now comes the even more important step of putting what you've read into action.

This is your time to become proactive, and get started on the road to physical strength. You can start today, or certainly tomorrow. There is no need to wait to buy equipment, because you can begin the basic exercises at home, with nothing more than some furniture, counters, or walls to lean on, and a mat or carpet to lie on and sit on.

Don't underestimate the muscle and strength-building potential of using only your own bodyweight for resistance. Recall that a push up lifts 65% of your weight, making it equal to a dumbbell or barbell chest press.

When you're ready, you may choose to use free weights—dumbbells especially—to intensify your training. Proceed as you've been instructed; gradually, with the understanding that you're in this for the long haul, and your investment of time and energy will earn big rewards in adding more life to your years, and more years to your life.

You also have the option to replicate weightlifting with elastic resistance bands. They're inexpensive and portable, and can also be used to intensify many of the basic exercises. You can also add isometrics to your workouts, to further tone and strengthen your muscles with just a few minutes of effort.

Succeed With Patience and Caution

You've seen the importance of rest repeated frequently in these pages, for the good reason that it's essential for the repair and rebuilding process of hypertrophy to gradually build muscle mass, strength, and endurance. Don't work the same muscles on consecutive days, and as a senior, it's best if you give your muscles two days to recover.

Remember the premise of the Hippocratic Oath, "First, do no harm." Take care of your joints by not pushing them too hard with weights that are too heavy. Patience is a virtue that is essential to your self protection. Remind yourself of how much time you'll lose if you overdo it by trying for immediate results. Strength building is a marathon, so pace yourself, and start out with lighter weights, and increase how much you're lifting gradually.

Pain is a warning that you need to stop before a joint, muscle, or tendon is injured. Strength training is strenuous if it is to be productive, but it should not cause pain. See a doctor or healthcare professional if it hurts, and get things checked out; you may need to modify how you work out, and possibly avoid certain exercises.

Your diet is a very important component of your health, as well as contributing to your strengthening progress. Avoid fad diets and commit to eating healthy and in moderation. The

Mediterranean diet that we've described is the one most medical professionals advocate. It's heart healthy, helps lower the risk of many diseases and chronic conditions, and it tastes great, so what's to lose?

Keep physically active as part of your lifestyle, because science is finding that being sedentary and sitting all day and evening can be injurious to your health. Walking is very beneficial, even if you can't commit to daily cardio workouts. Even standing when you work can do a lot of good.

Share the Spirit

If you have enjoyed reading *Strength Training for Seniors* and recognize its value in helping you to begin, or return to, a committed strength building program, please consider sharing your enthusiasm with others who can benefit.

You can do this by telling others who may be concerned about muscle loss, joint discomforts, bone porosity, and loss of energy and balance to read the book. You can also give the book a favorable review, which will encourage a wide readership.

In writing this book, my goal has been to help you, and every reader, to mature with improved strength, fitness, confidence, and dignity, rather than the declines most people associate with aging. Medical research is now finding that regular strength and cardio training keeps us not only physically stronger and healthier, but also slows or prevents cognitive declines.

In wishing you all the best in your self-improvement and well-being,

Mark Kemp

References

American Exercise Council. (2011, February 17). *Fitness for older adults — frequently asked questions.* https://www.acefitness.org/resources/everyone/blog/6734/fitness-for-older-adults-frequently-asked-questions/

Andrews, R. (2022). *All about strength training.* Precision Nutrition. https://www.precisionnutrition.com/all-about-strength-training

Better Health Channel. (2022). *Resistance training - preventing injury.* https://www.betterhealth.vic.gov.au/health/healthyliving/resistance-training-preventing-injury

California Mobility (2022). *21 Chair exercises for seniors: A comprehensive visual guide.* https://californiamobility.com/21-chair-exercises-for-seniors-visual-guide/

Canada's Food Guide. (2022, May 3). *Healthy eating for seniors.* https://food-guide.canada.ca/en/tips-for-healthy-eating/seniors/

Carlson, C. (2021, September 22). *20 Strength training moves to master for total body toning.* Women's Health.

https://www.womenshealthmag.com/fitness/g27393163/strength-training-exercises/

Chertoff, J. (2019, February 26). *Muscular hypertrophy and your workout.* Healthline. https://www.healthline.com/health/muscular-hypertrophy

Dellitt, J. (2022). *5 key strength training exercises for older adults.* Aaptiv. https://aaptiv.com/magazine/strength-training-for-older-adults-tips

Esposito, L., Fetters, K. (2020, September 30). *12 Best equipment-free strength exercises for older adults.* U.S. News & World Report. https://health.usnews.com/health-news/health-wellness/articles/best-equipment-free-strength-exercises-for-older-adults

Evolve. (2019, August 26). *Banded pull-through.* [YouTube Video]. https://youtu.be/RZ4HyxZBAdQ

Finlay, B. (2022). *How does your body move? Does the brain send it messages?* Cornell University. https://www.ccmr.cornell.edu/faqs/how-does-your-body-move-does-the-brain-send-it-messages/

Galic, B. (April 9, 2021). *The only 5 dumbbell exercises older adults need for total body strength.* Livestrong. https://www.livestrong.com/article/110562-dumbbell-exercises-seniors/

Gomez, J. (2020, May 23). *Strength training 101: How to get started.* Women's Health. https://www.womenshealthmag.com/fitness/a30522035/what-is-strength-training/

Gutman, A. (2020, November 6). *We asked strength coaches how to perform the most popular gym lifts at home — here's all the equipment you need to do them safely.* Insider. https://www.insider.com/guides/health/fitness/best-gym-lift-alternatives

Harvard Health Publishing. (2018, September 25). *8 Tips for safe and effective strength training.* https://www.health.harvard.edu/staying-healthy/8-tips-for-safe-and-effective-strength-training

Human Kinetics. (2022). *13 Benefits of strength training for people older than 50.* https://canada.humankinetics.com/blogs/articles/13-benefits-of-strength-training-for-people-older-than-50

ISSA. (2019, April 15). *The importance of strength training for seniors.* https://www.issaonline.com/blog/post/the-importance-of-strength-training-for-seniors

Johnson, J. (2022, January 22). *Our guide to the Mediterranean diet.* Medical News Today. https://www.medicalnewstoday.com/articles/324221

Jordan, M. (2021, March 29). *Joint pain isn't inevitable with age.* WebMD. https://www.webmd.com/osteoarthritis/features/joint-pain-management-age

Kernisan, L. (2022). *How to follow the Mediterranean diet for senior health & related research findings*. Better Health While Aging. https://betterhealthwhileaging.net/how-to-follow-mediterranean-diet-for-senior-health/

Kilroy, S. (2019, October 15). *Exercise plan for seniors*. Healthline. https://www.healthline.com/health/everyday-fitness/senior-workouts

Kita, P. (2020, May 19). *Fuel up, slim down, and build massive muscle with the new Men's Health strength diet*. Men's Health. https://www.menshealth.com/nutrition/a32584906/the-strength-diet/

Leeds, E. (2015, January 7). *Beginner's guide to muscle anatomy for strength training*. Total Gym. https://totalgymdirect.com/total-gym-blog/beginners-guide-to-muscle-anatomy

Lifeline. (2022). *14 Strength, flexibility, and balance exercises for seniors*. https://www.lifeline.com/blog/14-exercises-for-seniors-to-improve-strength-and-balance/

Living Maples. (2022, January 8). *The 7 best dumbbell exercises to boost senior's power*. https://livingmaples.com/mag/dumbbell-exercises-for-elderly

Mayo Clinic. (2022). *Aging: What to expect*. https://www.mayoclinic.org/healthy-lifestyle/healthy-aging/in-depth/aging/art-20046070

Mayo Clinic. (2022). *Strength training: Get stronger, leaner, healthier.* https://www.mayoclinic.org/healthy-lifestyle/fitness/in-depth/strength-training/art-20046670

MedlinePlus. (2022). *Aging changes in the heart and blood vessels.* https://medlineplus.gov/ency/article/004006.htm

MedlinePlus. (2022). *Nutrition for older adults.* https://medlineplus.gov/nutritionforolderadults.html

MyDr.com.au. (2019, January 23). *Physical activity benefits to your body.* https://www.mydr.com.au/sports-fitness/physical-activity-benefits-to-your-body/

National Institute on Aging. (2022). *Healthy meal planning: Tips for older adults.* https://www.nia.nih.gov/health/healthy-meal-planning-tips-older-adults

Nguyen, D. (2020, December 16). *Should elderly people engage in 1 rep maxes?* California Therapy Solutions. https://www.californiatherapysolutions.com/post/should-elderly-people-engage-in-1-rep-maxes

Reference. (2020, April 11). *How does age affect reflexes?* https://www.reference.com/science/age-affect-reflexes-6a50b9d46f186834

Rogers, P. (2019, November 26). *Repetition maximum for weight training.* Verywell Fit. https://www.verywellfit.com/what-is-repetition-maximum-and-1rm-3498379#:~:text=One%2DRepetition%20Maximum%20or%201RM&text=This%20indicates%20the%20heaviest%20weight,weight%20training%20for%20marking%20improvement

Seguin, R. et al. (2022). *Strength training for older adults*. CDC. https://www.cdc.gov/physicalactivity/downloads/growing_stronger.pdf

Semeco, A. (2021, December 14). *The top 10 benefits of regular exercise*. Healthline. https://www.healthline.com/nutrition/10-benefits-of-exercise

Silver Cuisine. (2017). *10 Foods to help seniors build strong muscles*. https://blog.silvercuisine.com/10-foods-to-help-seniors-build-strong-muscles/

Simon, G. (2022, January 8). *9 Dumbbell exercise for seniors - full body*. Heyday. https://heydaydo.com/dumbbell-exercises-seniors/

Sruthi, M. (2021, July 7). *What is good nutrition and a healthy diet?* MedicineNet. https://www.medicinenet.com/what_is_good_nutrition_and_a_healthy_diet/article.htm

Steinbaum, S. (2022, May 27). *What should we be putting in our bodies?* WebMD. https://blogs.webmd.com/heart-health/20220527/what-should-we-be-putting-in-our-bodies?ecd=wnl_faf_060622&ctr=wnl-faf-

060622_lead_cta&mb=MukfT6opS3AxbF5kSEwI0ng0WleHxvIqssh%40W36l9r4%3D

Vantage Aging. (2020, June 12). *10 Healthy eating tips for older adults*. https://vantageaging.org/blog/healthy-eating-tips-older-adults/

Volek, J. (2007, April). *Influence of nutrition on responses to resistance training*. National Institute of Health. https://pubmed.ncbi.nlm.nih.gov/15064597/

West Hartford Health & Rehabilitation Center. (2020, July 29). *The basics of joint health for seniors*. https://westhartfordhealth.com/news/senior-health/basics-joint-health/

York Fitness. (2022, May 31). *The top 5 benefits of strength training for seniors*. https://yorkfitness.com/blogs/articles/the-top-5-benefits-of-strength-training-for-seniors

Image References

Ready Made. (2020, May 14). *Healthy ingredients composition*. [Image]. Pexels. https://www.pexels.com/photo/healthy-ingredients-composition-of-vegetables-near-wine-and-utensils-on-table-in-kitchen-3850884/

Tentis, D. (2018, July 10) *Vegetable salad with wheat bread*. [Image]. Pexels. https://www.pexels.com/photo/vegetable-salad-with-wheat-bread-on-the-side-1213710/

Tentis, D. (2017, December 10). *Cooked meal with vegetables*. [Image]. Pexels. https://www.pexels.com/photo/cooked-meat-with-vegetables-725991/

Printed in Great Britain
by Amazon